MRI in Clinical Practice

MRI in Clinical Practice

Gary Liney

With 62 Figures

Springer

Gary Liney, PhD, SRCS
MRI Lecturer
University of Hull
Centre for MR Investigations
Hull Royal Infirmary
Hull
UK

British Library Cataloguing in Publication Data
A catalogue record for this book is available from the British Library

Library of Congress Control Number: 2005930807

ISBN-10: 1-84628-161-X e-ISBN 1-84628-162-8 Printed on acid-free paper
ISBN-13: 978-1-84628-161-7

Printed in Singapore (BS/KYO)

9 8 7 6 5 4 3 2 1

Springer Science+Business Media
springeronline.com

Dedication

For Emma and my kids, David, Rebecca, and Matthew

Tomorrow is a new day

English Proverb

Contents

Introduction

When I was asked to write this book, my first thought was how was I going to improve on what was already out there? There are literally dozens of enormous volumes covering the everexpanding field of MRI. This rather more concise effort attempts to pull together lots of vital information and condense it down into a simple-to-follow guide. It will be useful for trainees and experienced professionals alike.

Part I includes sections covering the basic physical principles behind MRI, quality assurance, up-to-date safety guidelines, and a useful gallery of image artifacts. Part II covers six anatomical sections, illustrating the main areas where MRI is being exploited today, describing both its routine and advanced utilization.

The book has been written at a time when more and more sites move from 1.5 to 3.0 Tesla, and the important issues concerning this transition are highlighted. Interspersed throughout the book you will also find some useful hints and tips. The book concludes with an Appendix, including a glossary of the everincreasing (and often confusing) pulse sequence acronyms.

Although not intended to replace many of the existing texts, it nevertheless should be a first stop for those seeking clarification or some revision!

Gary Liney
February 2006

The front cover illustrates the use of MRI "from head to toe", showing a 3D reconstruction of the author's brain, a MIP renal angiogram, and a T_1-weighted image of a right foot. All images in this book were acquired at Hull Royal Infirmary, England, using 1.5 Tesla Philips Intera, 1.5 Tesla, and 3.0 Tesla GE Signa scanners.

Acknowledgments

I am particularly grateful to the following people: Chris Beadle (volunteer images in 3.1), Martin Pickles (some of the "Top Tips" and proofreading the anatomical sections), Dr. Muthyala Sreenivas (gynecology), Dr. David Nag (musculoskeletal), and Roberto Garcia-Alvarez (Figures 5.5 and 5.7).

Thanks also to the Centre for MR Investigations, Hull Royal Infirmary, and Yorkshire Cancer Research.

Part I

Chapter 1
The Basics

1.1 SOME MR PHYSICS

Magnetic Moment and Spin

The fundamental concept behind MRI is the spinning nuclear charge, which produces a tiny magnetic field called a magnetic moment. This field can be treated as a tiny bar magnet with a north–south direction. The simplest and most useful nucleus to consider is that of the hydrogen atom, naturally abundant in the human body and comprising a single proton. In the normal environment, the random orientation of millions of these spins results in no net magnetic field. However, the situation changes when these spins are placed in a strong external magnetic field such as that of the scanner, referred to as B_0. The spins now align themselves in given directions, but rather than simply turning, their angular momentum causes the spins to precess at a certain frequency. This characteristic frequency (ω_0) is given by the Larmor equation:

$$\omega_0 = \gamma B_0,$$

where γ is a constant called the *magnetogyric ratio* (sometimes called the gyromagnetic ratio).

❖ How Strong is the MRI Scanner?
A typical clinical scanner has a magnetic field of 1.5 Tesla. To put this into perspective, the Earth's field is approximately 0.5 Gauss (1 T = 10,000 G), meaning the scanner is thirty thousand times stronger!

Quantum Physics

According to the laws of quantum physics, the spin property of a nucleus can only be a discrete value, represented by the spin quantum number (I). For nuclei to be "MR visible" the value of this number is nonzero. The number of possible spin energy states in an external magnetic field is given by $2I + 1$. In the case of a proton, I is equal to $^1/_2$, meaning there are two such states, *spin-up* and *spin-down*. The spin-up state is the lowest energy state and corresponds to alignment along the direction of B_0. The higher energy spin-down state corresponds to antiparallel alignment. At thermal equilibrium (i.e., normal room temperature), there are slightly more spins in the lower state. This tiny majority produces a small net magnetic field, the *net magnetization* M_0, in the direction of B_0 (Figure 1.1(a)).

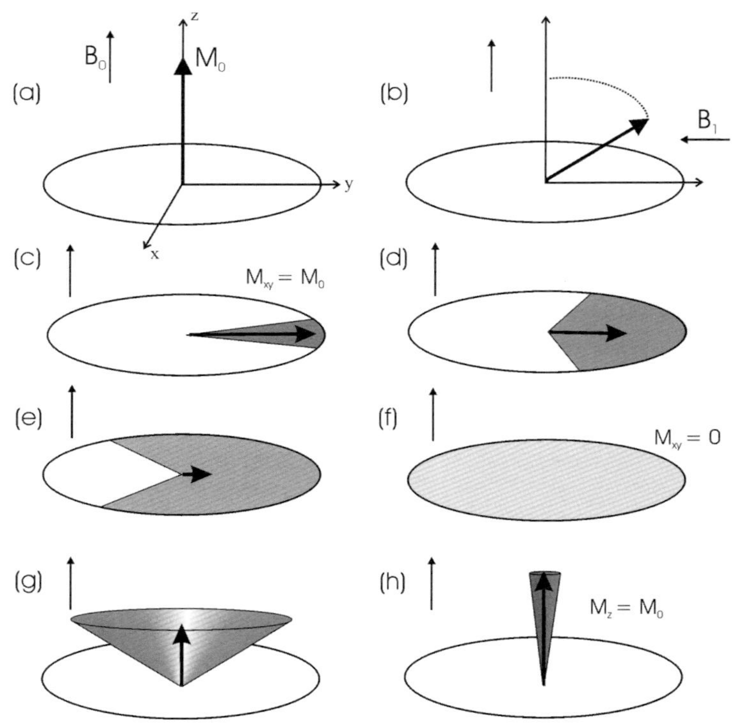

FIGURE 1.1. (a) to (h) Relaxation mechanisms.

- ❖ Which Nuclei are MR Visible?
  The nuclei of the following atoms are all MR visible ($I \neq 0$) and are often used in MRI and MRS. They are (in order of sensitivity): ^{1}H, ^{13}C, ^{19}F, ^{23}Na, and ^{31}P (see also Chapters 7 and 9 for applications).

Application of the B$_1$ Field

In order to observe this net effect (M_0), a second field called B_1 is introduced. This field must have two important characteristics: first it has to act in a perpendicular direction to B_0, and second it must be applied at the resonant frequency of the spins, which for the proton is in the radio-frequency (RF) range. The spins begin to precess about this second field, resulting in a spiraling motion away from the B_0 direction. This can be simplified by adopting the so-called *rotating frame of reference*, the situation as observed from the spins. In this case, the overall effect is to turn the net magnetization towards the transverse plane (xy) as shown in Figure 1.1(b). If the B_1 field is applied sufficiently long enough, the magnetization ends up in the xy-plane. This application of the B_1 field is described as an *excitation pulse*, and in this case a pulse with a 90° (π/2 radians) flip angle has been used. The transverse component of magnetization (M_{xy}) is now equal to M_0, and is detected in a receiver coil placed in the xy-plane (Figure 1.1(c)).

Relaxation

Once the RF field has been switched off the spins begin to return to the original equilibrium situation with the net magnetization aligned with B_0. There are two mechanisms that occur to make this happen. First the individual spins begin to experience slightly different magnetic fields due to the inhomogeneity of the scanner and also interactions between spins. These differences in field result in different precessional frequencies as governed by the Larmor equation. The spins begin to spread out or dephase in the xy-plane (Figure 1.1(c) to (f)) resulting in a rapid decay of the signal M_{xy} to zero. This is known as *transverse relaxation* (or T_2*) and the characteristic signal is called the *free induction decay* or FID.

Loss of energy to the spin-lattice forces the recovery of the magnetization along the z-direction. This is known as T_1 *relaxation* and as the spins return to the original alignment with B_0, the z or longitudinal component of the magnetization M_z, increases from zero to its maximum value M_0 (Figure 1.1(g), (h)).

The time allowed for this recovery is the repetition time (*TR*), discussed in detail later on.

Spin-Echo

A second important concept in MRI is the spin-echo (illustrated in Figure 1.2). Some of the decaying FID may be recovered by using a *refocusing pulse*. This is a second application of B_1, which acts to turn the spins 180° so that the phases are reversed. In Figure 1.2, T_2* decay occurs from (a) to (c). At time $t = TE/2$ (d) the refocusing pulse is applied in the *xy*-plane. Note that this pulse can be applied along either the *x*-direction, ((d) to (f)) or the *y*-direction ((g) to (i)). In either case, the faster spins (yellow)

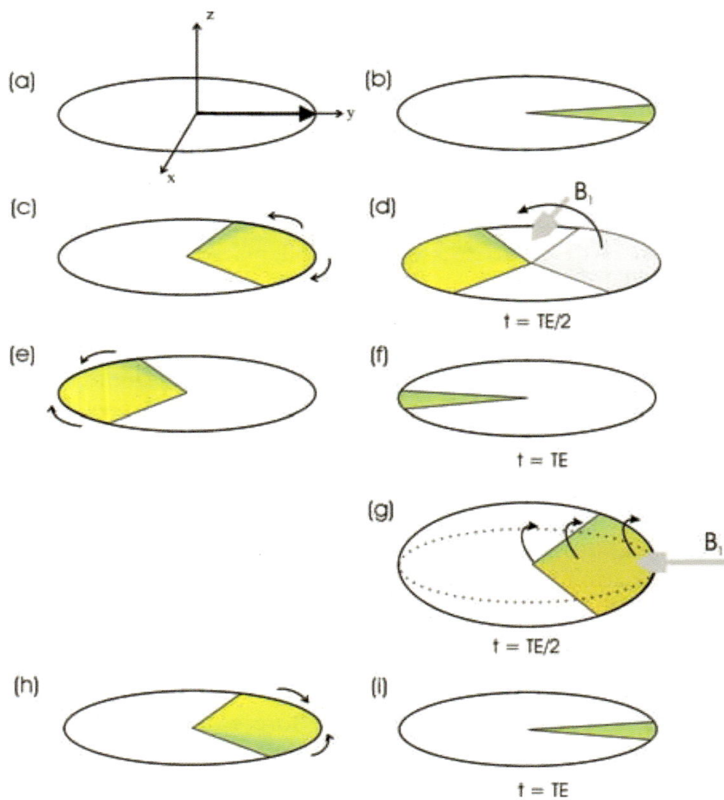

FIGURE 1.2. Formation of a spin-echo.

are now behind the slower spins (green). After the same period of time the faster spins have caught up and a signal echo will be produced at time *TE*. This signal will have recovered losses due to T_2* effects but natural spin–spin (T_2) losses will not be recovered. The signal is now said to be T_2-weighted.

Other Echoes

A *Hahn echo* utilizes two RF pulses of arbitrary flip angles. For the maximum signal, 90° and 180° pulses must be employed in the manner described above; however, any two RF pulses will produce a spin-echo.

A *gradient-echo*, discussed in Section 1.3, is produced by the reversal of a magnetic field gradient, and does not require a refocusing pulse.

A *stimulated echo* is created from the application of at least three RF pulses. It should be noted that there will also be additional spin-echoes produced from each possible combination of RF pairs. A stimulated echo is often an unwanted side effect in a multipulse sequence and is often deliberately removed using crusher gradients. A stimulated echo is used in the STEAM sequence in spectroscopy (Section 1.3).

Chemical Shift

The chemical shift effect is fundamental to MR spectroscopy (MRS). The nature of the effect is to produce a change in resonant frequency for nuclei of the same type attached to different chemical species. It is due to variations in surrounding electron clouds of neighboring atoms, which shield nuclei from the main magnetic field. The resulting difference (or shift) in frequency can be used to identify the presence of important metabolites in the body.

Fat Suppression

The bulk of the MR signal in the human body arises from protons in either water or fat molecules. In certain applications it is best to suppress the fat signal and there are several ways this is achieved.

Short Tau Inversion Recovery (STIR)

This method exploits the different T_1 relaxation times of fat and water and is illustrated in Figure 1.3, with the fat signal shown as a double-headed arrow (a). First, an inversion pulse (180° flip angle, (b)) is used to rotate the fat and water signals along the $-z$-direction. (c) The two signals recover along the z-direction, the

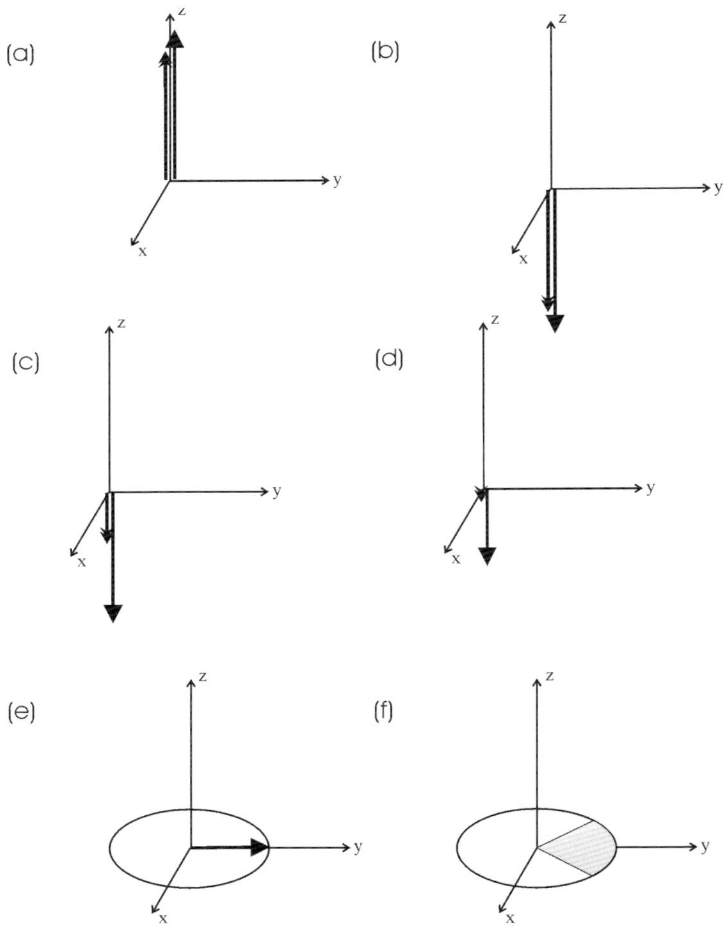

FIGURE 1.3. (a) to (f) Short T_1 inversion recovery for fat suppression.

fat recovering more quickly owing to a shorter T_1. At the null point (d), the fat magnetization has a zero component in this direction. (e) Now a 90° pulse (sometimes called an inspection pulse) is used to flip the spins into the transverse plane, and only water contributes to the measured signal which then proceeds to dephase as normal (f). The appropriate time interval (200 ms at

1.5 Tesla), is referred to by the Greek symbol tau, τ. The disadvantage of this method is that this time interval is fixed, and hence the image contrast cannot be altered.

> Top Tip! Perform any inversion-prepared sequences (such as STIR or FLAIR) prior to using contrast agents as the inversion times will alter following T_1 enhancement.

Chemical Selective Saturation (CHESS)
In this case it is the chemical shift between the fat and water protons that is exploited. At 1.5 Tesla the difference in resonance is approximately 220 Hz. This means that a narrow bandwidth RF pulse centered on the appropriate resonance can affect either the fat or water as required. In the commonly used CHESS method (shown in Figure 1.4), the fat pulse is turned slightly into the $-z$-direction (b), where it is dephased by gradients (c). By the time the imaging sequence begins (d), there is no fat signal and the water peak is only imaged.

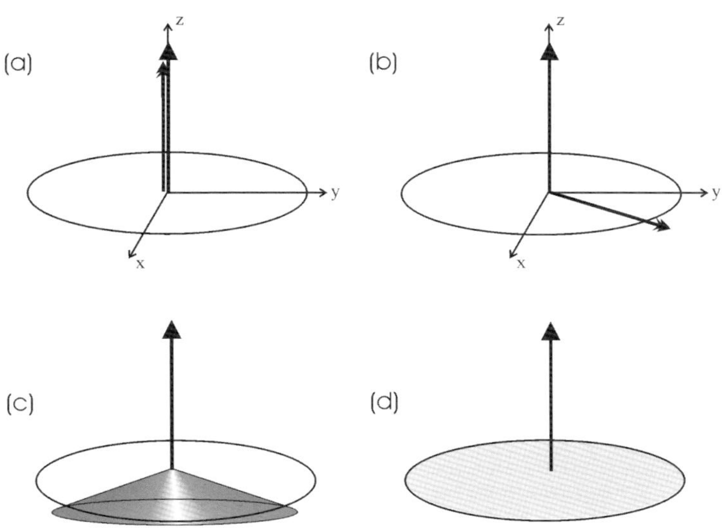

FIGURE 1.4. (a) to (d) Frequency (chemical) selective fat suppression.

> Top Tip! Use of a localized volume shim during pre-scan will improve image quality in sequences that rely on good homogeneity (e.g., CHESS and gradient-echo).

Binomial Pulse Method

The resonant frequency differences described above cause a phase shift to accrue between fat and water. A *binomial* excitation pulse may be used, which consists of splitting the normal 90° flip angle into separate pulses, which follow a binomial series. In the case shown in Figure 1.5, a 1:–1 pulse is used, or two pulses with angles of 45° and –45°. The first pulse turns both water and fat to make a 45° angle with the *z*-direction as shown in (b). A period of time is observed so that the faster precessing water peak is completely out of phase with the fat peak (c). A –45° pulse (d) is then applied which turns the fat peak into the transverse plane and the water returns back along the *z*-direction and is available for subsequent imaging.

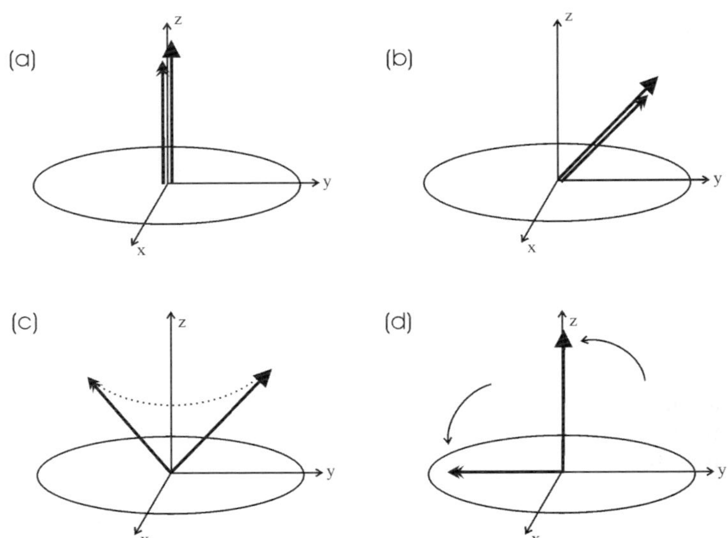

FIGURE 1.5. (a) to (d) Use of a binomial pulse in selective excitation.

1.2 IMAGE FORMATION

Contrast Weighting

One of the main advantages of MRI over other imaging modalities such as CT is its excellent soft-tissue contrast, which can be widely manipulated. The signal measured will depend on the number of spins present (the proton density, PD), as well as their T_1 and T_2 relaxation times. By altering the sequence timings (*TE* and *TR*) and sometimes the flip angles too, the image contrast can be weighted so that one of these effects predominates, although all maintain a contribution.

For example, to produce a T_2-weighted image the T_1 differences should be minimized by using a short *TR* and acquiring the echo late-on, that is, a long *TE*. To acquire T_1-weighting in the image, the opposite argument applies: a short *TE* will reduce the effects of T_2-weighting, whereas a long *TR* will enhance the differences in T_1 relaxation times. With both T_1 and T_2 effects minimized the contrast will be essentially due to the (proton) density of spins and achieved using a short *TE* and a long *TR*.

So to summarize:

- T_2-weighting: long *TE* and long *TR* (e.g., >100 ms/ >3 s)
- T_1-weighting: short *TE* and short *TR* (e.g., <<50 ms/<<500 ms)
- *PD*-weighting: short *TE* and long *TR*

Slice Selection

The signal recorded thus far has been from the entire sensitive volume of the (RF) receiver coil. In order to form an image, the signal must be spatially discriminated. This is first achieved using a method known as slice selection, whereby only a finite section of spins (the image slice) is excited into the transverse plane. First, a *gradient*, or a linear change in the B_0 field, is created along the slice direction causing the frequency of the spins to also change in this direction. A specially shaped RF pulse, called a *sinc pulse*, containing a bandwidth of frequencies will then excite only the spins at corresponding resonance. This is illustrated in Figure 1.6 (left), in the case of two cylinders whose long axes are along the *z*-direction. A cross-section is to be selectively excited in this direction by first turning on the gradient G_z. The resulting change in precessional frequency means a 90° pulse with a bandwidth equal to $\pm\,\Delta\omega$ will act on this small section of spins only. The width and location of the slice can be altered by changing the gradient and the bandwidth. Due to practical constraints the sinc pulse has to be truncated so that the profile is no longer

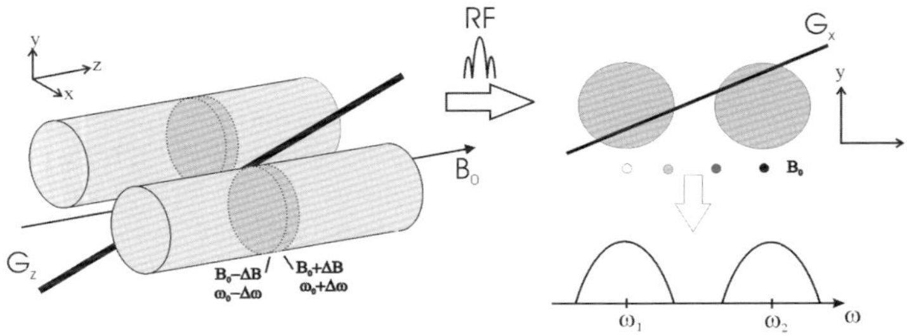

FIGURE 1.6. Example of slice-selection (left) and frequency encoding (right).

a perfect square, leading to cross-excitation of adjacent spins (see also Chapter 3).

> Top Tip! To improve imaging coverage without adding slices or increasing thickness, consider increasing the slice gap instead. Some scanners also permit the use of slice offsets.

Frequency and Phase Encoding

Two additional gradients are required to spatially encode the image in the remaining two dimensions. The first gradient is applied at the time of signal measurement, called the *read* or *frequency-encoding gradient*. This changes the frequency along the direction of the gradient so that the frequency differences in the final signal correspond linearly with spatial location. In Figure 1.6, this has been done in the x-direction; the B_0 field and therefore the precessional frequency increases along x (indicated by increasingly dark circles), resulting in two spatially distinct signals about ω_1 and ω_2.

The final dimension cannot be encoded by changes of frequency: there would always be ambiguously assigned pixels that could not be distinguished. For the remaining direction, the signal is encoded by changes of phase. This is done by applying the gradient at the start of the sequence and repeating it many times, each with a different increment of the gradient amplitude. The number of pixels (image *matrix*) in this direction determines the number of phase-encoding steps required.

2D and 3D Imaging

Multiple slice imaging is achieved by utilizing the period between the echo collection and before the next excitation pulse (*TR–TE*, or the *dead time*) to excite adjacent slices. To account for imperfect excitation profiles, slices are usually acquired with an interslice gap or alternatively, in an interleaved fashion, with the "odd" slices imaged prior to the "even" slices being acquired.

In 3D imaging, phase encoding is also utilized in the through-plane direction. This improves the spatial resolution in this dimension, from what can be achieved with slice-selection (typically 2–5 mm), to that of the in-plane dimensions (<1 mm). As a result the imaging voxels are more isotropic and the three-dimensional visualization and reconstruction of the data are much better. The scan time increases by a factor equal to the number of phase encodings in the third dimension but the increased number of signal measurements means that signal-to-noise is inherently better.

Fourier Transformation

Fourier transformation (FT) permits a time-varying signal to be decomposed into a series of sinusoidal waveforms each with different amplitude (a), phase (φ), and frequency (ω). The FT of a time-varying signal $S(t)$ is given by:

$$S(t) = a_0 + a_1\sin(\omega_1 t + \varphi_1) + a_2\sin(\omega_2 t + \varphi_2) + \ldots a_n\sin(\omega_n t + \varphi_n).$$

FT is used in MRI to decode the detected signal and spatially assign each pixel row and column in the final image.

Contrast Agents

The different tissue signals within an image can be further manipulated by using exogenous contrast agents. By far the most common are the *gadolinium*-based agents, which are injected intravenously and followed with a saline flush to ensure delivery. Gadolinium is a paramagnetic ion, with a high relaxivity; that is, it disturbs the local magnetic field of nearby protons and results in a shortening of T_1 and T_2 relaxation times. It has to be chelated to another molecule, called a ligand, to ensure it is excreted. Currently four gadolinium-chelates are in widespread clinical use. These are given below with the chemical names in brackets and trade names in italics:

- Gadopentetate dimeglumine (Gd-DTPA), *Magnevist*
- Gadoteridol (Gd-HP-DO3A), *ProHance*

- Gadodiamide (Gd-DTPA-BMA), *Omniscan*
- Gadoterate meglumine (Gd-DOTA), *Dotarem*

(Another agent, Gadovist, is discussed in MRA section.)

Although the T_1 and T_2 relaxivity of these agents is similar, T_1 effects dominate at low concentrations due to the inherently longer tissue T_1 values. In a T_1-weighted image the agents produce an increase in signal intensity. They are often used in cancer, as the increased blood supply to rapidly growing tumors preferentially takes up the agent and improves tumor conspicuity.

Other categories of contrast agents are as follows.

Blood Pool Agents

The T_1-shortening effect may be used to directly image vasculature in a technique known as *contrast-enhanced MR angiography* (CE-MRA). Unfortunately the extracellular nature of most agents renders them a short half-life in the blood and causes unwanted background tissue enhancement. Specific blood pool agents are so called because they reversibly bind to blood protein albumin (e.g., AngioMARK, Multihance), which prolongs their stay in the vascular tree.

Targeted Agents

Some agents may be described as targeted or organ specific. Common examples of these include those that are taken up by the liver, improving the visualization of liver lesions. Gadolinium or manganese-based agents as well as super-paramagnetic iron oxides (SPIO) are all used to image the liver (see Chapter 7). Depending on their particle size, ultrasmall versions (USPIO) may also be used to image the lymph nodes.

Other

Enteral agents are contrast agents that are administered orally or rectally in order to image the bowel, producing either positive or negative enhancement. Some natural substances (e.g., blueberry juice) may also be given as contrast. Finally, gases may be used for ventilation imaging of the lung. More often than not these are *hyperpolarized gases* (helium or xenon) but gadolinium-based aerosols also exist.

A full list of contrast agents either in common use or currently undergoing clinical trials is given in Appendix A2.1.

k-Space Made Simple

Figure 1.7 (right) shows the *k*-space representation of the image on the left. Put simply, *k*-space is an array of numbers the FT of

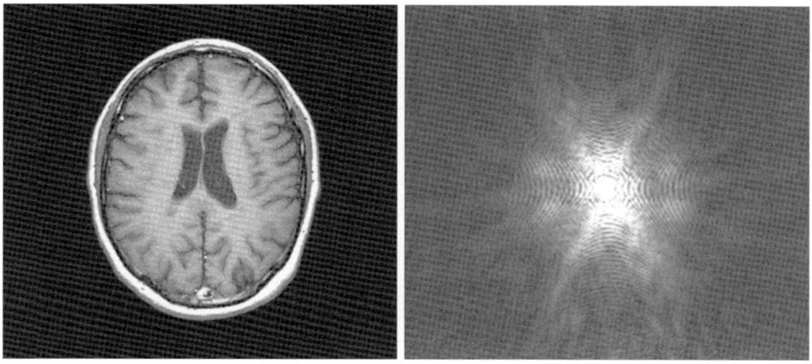

FIGURE 1.7. An image (left) and its corresponding representation in *k*-space (right).

which produces the MR image. *k*-space is often represented as a diagram with the *x*- and *y*-axis to illustrate the acquisition of MR data, although elements between the image-space and *k*-space do not correspond one-to-one. Each data point in *k*-space contains information about every pixel in the image.

A row of *k*-space corresponds to the echo data collected with each application of the phase-encoding gradient. To produce an image, the full area of *k*-space must be traversed. Data near the center of *k*-space correspond to small amplitudes of the phase-encoding gradient, and the bulk of the image signal. Towards the edges of *k*-space, data are acquired with high phase-encoding amplitudes, corresponding to low signal but high spatial detail.

❖ What is the "*k*" in *k*-space?
k actually refers to the wave-number, or the number of wave cycles per unit distance. It is related to the application of imaging gradients by $k = \gamma Gt$, where G and t are the amplitude and duration of the gradient, respectively. The product Gt is the area of the gradient in a pulse sequence diagram (discussed next).

1.3 PULSE SEQUENCES

Pulse Sequence Diagrams

A pulse sequence diagram is a representation of the RF pulses and gradients that are necessary to acquire the image. Usually a separate row is used to represent the action of the RF pulses, each orthogonal gradient (G_S, G_P, and G_F for slice, phase, and frequency encoding), and the signal produced over the time of one repetition (*TR*). The gradients are illustrated by rectangles, the area of which indicates their amplitude and duration. By convention, a positive gradient appears above the baseline, and a negative gradient is drawn below it.

Spin-echo

The generic spin-echo sequence is shown in Figure 1.8. Note the negative gradients (called dephasing lobes) on G_s and G_F. These ensure that the spins are rephased at the end of slice selection and at the center of the echo, respectively. The diagram represents just one repetition of the full sequence. To acquire all the image data, the pulse sequence is repeated with a different amplitude of the phase-encoding gradient (indicated by multiple lines on G_P).

The total scan time is therefore given by

$$N_P \times TR \times N_A,$$

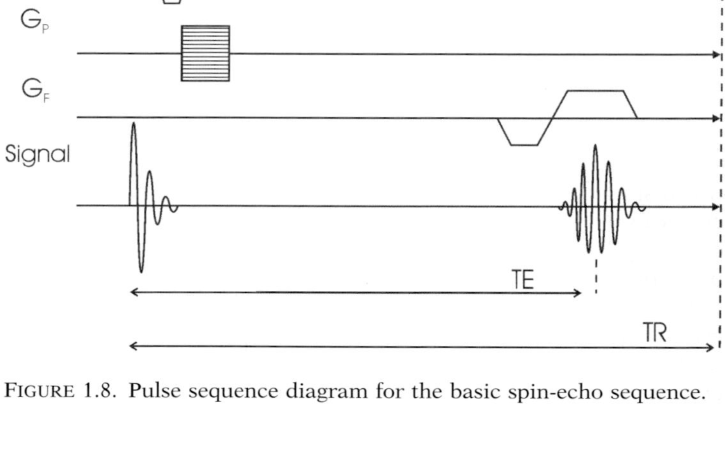

FIGURE 1.8. Pulse sequence diagram for the basic spin-echo sequence.

where N_P is the number of phase encoding steps and N_A is the number of signal averages employed (see Section 3.1, Signal Averaging).

Multiple Spin-echo

A modification to this sequence is the multiple spin-echo (MSE). In this case more than one refocusing pulse is used to produce multiple echoes at various *TE*s. This produces images with a variety of weightings; for example, the early echo may have proton-density-like contrast and subsequent echoes will have more T_2-weighting. Alternatively it may be used to measure T_2 (CPMG sequence).

Gradient-echo

A gradient-echo, GRE, (also known as a *field-echo* or *gradient-recalled echo*) is produced whenever the amplitude of a gradient is reversed (Figure 1.9). In this case there is no need for a 180° refocusing pulse, which means that the minimum *TR* is much shorter than in the spin-echo, giving the advantage of increased speed. For reduced *TR*s ($TR \ll T_1$) it is efficient to use a small flip angle (indicated by $\alpha°$) to maintain significant magnetization in the transverse plane while allowing for the small period of recovery in the longitudinal direction. The optimum angle, called the *Ernst angle*, is given by:

$$\cos\alpha_E = \exp(-TR/T_1)$$

For long values of *TR* ($TR \gg T_1$), the optimum flip angle is 90° as in the case of a spin-echo.

The absence of the phase refocusing means that the gradient-echo is inherently T_2* weighted and as such, the sequence is prone to artifacts from inhomogeneities such as susceptibility effects (discussed in Section 3.2).

Fast Spin-echo

At first glance the fast spin-echo (FSE) sequence (also known as turbo spin-echo) looks like the MSE (Figure 1.10). However, on closer examination it can be seen that there are different phase-encoding steps for each echo. This means that the echoes can be used together to produce a single image more quickly. The reduction in scan time is given by the total number of echoes (*echo train length* or turbo factor). The overall effective *TE* is the time of the central echo. Use of long echo trains or large echo spacing can result in blurred images.

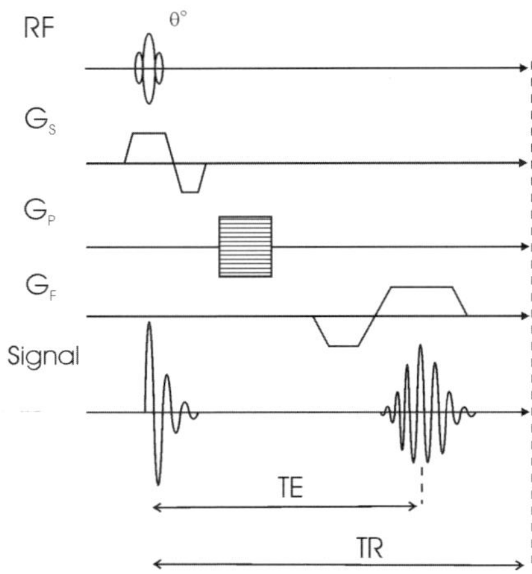

FIGURE 1.9. Pulse sequence diagram for the gradient-echo sequence.

> Top Tip! For T_1-weighted FSE scans limit the echo train length to 3 or 5 to prevent blurring.

EPI

Echo planar imaging (EPI), Figure 1.11, is a gradient-intensive sequence capable of acquiring all the necessary phase-encoding steps in a single *TR* (*single shot*), producing images at a rate of a few milliseconds per slice. Usually a reduced resolution is acquired (typically 64 or 128 matrix). It is useful whenever short image times are needed, for example pediatric imaging and fMRI (Section 5.3).

MRS Localization

Many different MRS sequences are used to localize the desired volume of interest in either a single or multivoxel technique. The two most commonly employed sequences are STEAM and PRESS, which utilize slice selection in each orthogonal direction to measure either a stimulated echo or a spin-echo from the intersected volume of interest (VOI). The volume may be subdivided using phase encoding in two or three dimensions to obtain spectra from smaller voxels. Metabolic concentrations are several orders of magnitude smaller than water and fat meaning that

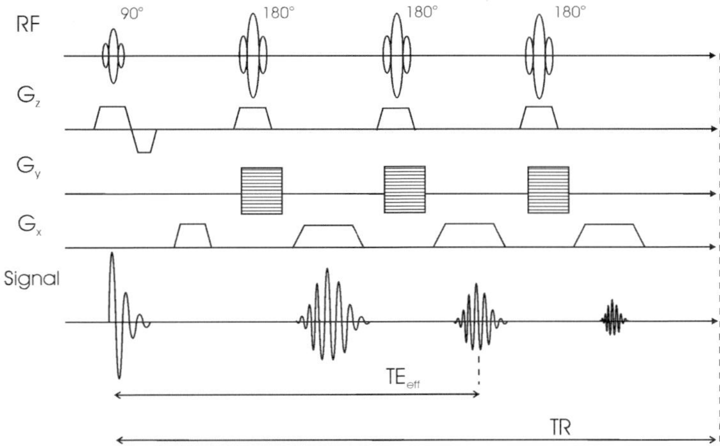

FIGURE 1.10. Pulse sequence diagram for the fast spin-echo sequence.

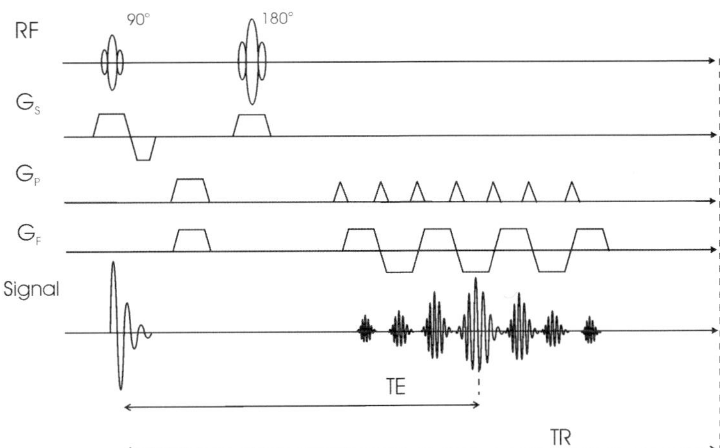

FIGURE 1.11. Pulse sequence diagram for the echo planar imaging sequence.

these larger peaks need to be removed from the spectrum. Water suppression is achieved using chemical shift selective (CHESS) pulses, and lipid (fat) contamination is reduced by using outer volume saturation bands (see below). Signal-to-noise requirements mean that spatial resolution is much worse than in imaging, and currently a 1 cm^3 voxel size is considered acceptable.

Other Notable Sequences

For completeness here are a few brief comments on other types of sequences you may come across.

Steady-state

A steady-state sequence maintains a transverse magnetization by using repetitive RF pulses with a very short *TR* so that effectively, $TR << T_2$. A continuous train of FID and spin-echo signals are produced, either of which may be sampled. Examples of this type of sequence include GRASS and FISP, which employ phase rewinding and are sometimes referred to as refocused steady-state. Balanced-gradient sequences, in which the FID and echo coincide, include FIESTA and TrueFISP.

Driven Equilibrium

In a driven equilibrium sequence, a –90° pulse is used to force the transverse magnetization to return quickly along the z-direction rather than waiting for T_1 recovery. This ensures a high fluid signal with reduced scan times. Examples of this type of sequence include DRIVE and FRFSE.

Magnetization Transfer (MT) Imaging

This refers to off-resonance RF pulses that are used to saturate signal from large macromolecules such as proteins. The effect on mobile water protons produces a new type of image contrast and has been used in demyelination, in MRA to improve vessel visualization, and also in contrast-enhancement studies.

Pre-scan and Localizer

The pre-scan is usually an automatic routine performed by the scanner prior to image acquisition. During this period the coil is tuned to the appropriate resonant frequency, and the receiver and transmitter gains are adjusted accordingly. Failure to do this results in a general degradation of image quality (also see Section 3.2, Over-ranging Artifact). The homogeneity of the prescribed volume can also be improved by *shimming* (see Section 1.4). Additional steps such as water suppression for MRS may be performed. Sometimes the procedure will fail, that is, not achieve a default tolerance and the pre-scan must be performed manually.

The first images in an examination are the *localizer* (or *scout*) images, which are a rapidly collected set of images from which subsequent scans are prescribed. On older systems the localizer is usually only available in a single plane, whereas modern scanners typically acquire this in all three planes.

Saturation Bands

These involve the application of slice-selection and dephasing gradients to remove the signal contribution from specific user-defined volumes of tissue. It is useful to eliminate unwanted signal contributions, for example, flow artifacts or contamination from outside MRS voxels.

Spoiling

Transverse magnetization at the end of each *TR* may be actively destroyed by using gradient or RF spoiling. In some rapid gradient-echo sequences (e.g., FLASH and FSPGR), spoiling is used to avoid a steady-state buildup.

Partial *k*-Space

There are several imaging techniques that only acquire part of *k*-space in order to speed up imaging time, either by reducing the number of phase-encoding steps or measuring only half of the echo. Sequences may acquire as little as half of *k*-space and fill in the missing data due to the inherent conjugate symmetry of *k*-space: the mirrored locations through the origin are identical. Keyhole imaging, is another example of partially filling *k*-space to improve imaging speed (see Section 9.3).

A slightly different approach is used in *parallel imaging*. In this case lines of *k*-space are missed out altogether and these data are replaced by using information from the sensitivity profiles of coil elements.

In all cases speed is traded off for poorer image quality and reduced signal-to-noise.

❖ What is Parallel Imaging?
This is a technique for speeding up scan times by replacing some of the time-consuming gradient

encoding steps with "coil encoding". Missing lines of *k*-space are reconstructed from combinations of separate coil signals in multicoil arrays. This reconstruction can occur in *k*-space (SMASH, GRAPPA) or by unwrapping signals in image-space (SENSE). The maximum speed-up factor is given by the number of separate coil elements. Currently clinical scanners are limited to factors of between 2 and 4.

1.4 A WORD ON HARDWARE

Magnets

Nearly all clinical scanners are *superconducting* magnets with a horizontal bore design. These are electromagnets that are made from superconducting alloys such as niobium–titanium. To achieve superconductivity and therefore zero electrical resistance they need to be cooled below a certain critical temperature. This is achieved using liquid helium, which surrounds the magnet windings in the cryostat, and needs to be replenished regularly. Lower field systems may be resistive electromagnets and some earlier machines even used permanent magnetic cores.

Open design magnets permit interventional work during scanning and reduce claustrophobia. However, this is becoming less of an issue with modern wide, short bore scanners. Even at 3.0 Tesla the bore can be reduced to lengths much shorter than the "tunnels" that were produced only a few years ago. The system in Figure 1.12, with a bore length of just 1.4 m, claims to be the world's shortest bore at 1.5 Tesla.

The homogeneity of the main field is specified by its *DSV* or the diameter of a spherical volume centered about the magnet isocenter, within which the field varies the least. A "40 cm DSV of 1 ppm" means that the field varies by no more than 1 Hz per 10^6 Hz in any 20 cm distance from the center. Open and short bore designs can be expected to be less homogeneous than their longer closed bore counterparts. The homogeneity of the magnet is adjusted through the process of shimming. Some passive shimming is done at the time of manufacture by fixing sheets of metal at certain points. Active shimming may be done prior to scanning by adjusting currents in an additional set of magnet windings.

The magnet has to be shielded in order to confine the fringe field to a practical distance. In the earliest scanners, passive shielding was used whereby lumps of steel would be strategically

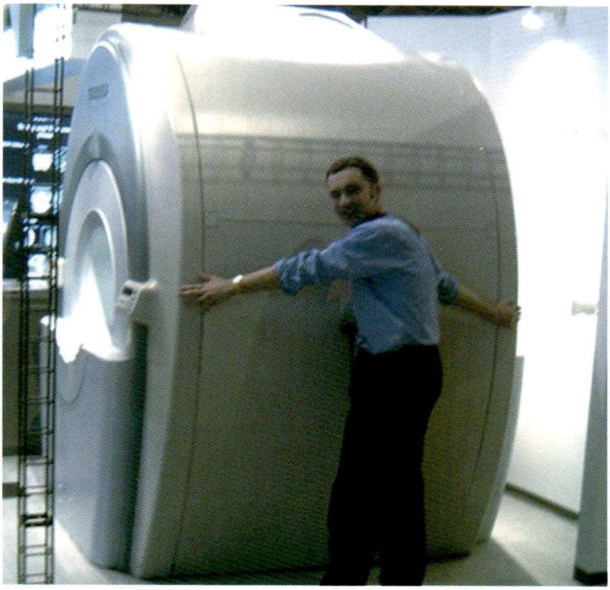

FIGURE 1.12. The author demonstrates the length of this short bore scanner.

placed in the scanner room. Nowadays, all clinical scanners are *actively shielded*, utilizing opposite flowing current in external windings to counteract the B_0 field.

The magnet itself is housed in a specially constructed room with copper lining the walls and ceiling to create what is known as a *Faraday cage*. This ensures that extraneous RF cannot penetrate into the room thus preventing artifacts (see Section 3.2, RF Artifact).

Gradients

Additional coils are needed within the magnet to provide the gradients in each orthogonal direction. A Maxwell pair is used to provide the z-direction gradient, whereas two sets of Golay coils are needed for the x- and y-directions.

The rapidly changing fields of the gradients induce oscillating eddy currents and, as a result, magnetic fields in the surrounding conductors. These produce distortions in the image and require the gradients themselves to be shielded in a similar manner to the main field.

Gradient performance is specified in terms of *slew rate*, or the maximum amplitude divided by the *rise time* (time taken to switch from zero to maximum value). A typical modern scanner may have an amplitude of 40 m*T*/m and rise time of 200 μs giving a slew rate of 200 *T*/ms.

RF Coils

To provide the B_1 field necessary for transmission and reception, RF coils are required, either working separately or as combined transceivers. Coils are designed to be appropriately sized for the anatomy under examination, which ensures optimum signal-to-noise. Image quality is further influenced by the transmission/reception profile of the coil (see Section 3.1, RF Coil).

The simplest design consists of a single loop of wire for use as a *surface coil*, giving excellent signal near the coil but rapidly dropping off farther away. More complicated designs such as those used in the head and body coils, produce lower signal but are more homogeneous.

Surface coils may be combined to form phased arrays. These have the advantage of excellent signal with improved coverage. Careful consideration has to be made concerning the overlap of the individual coil elements.

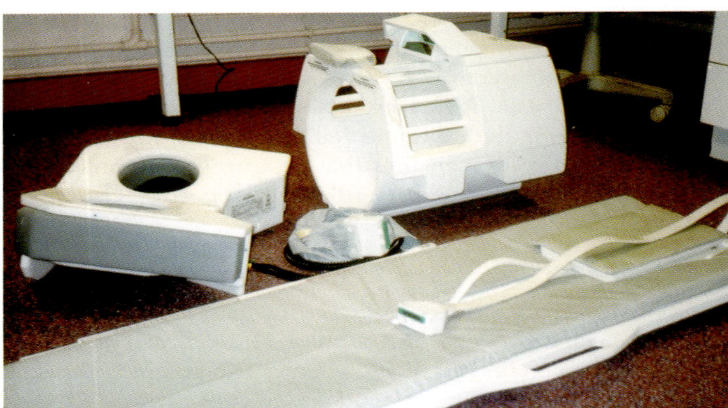

FIGURE 1.13. A selection of RF coils (bottom) pelvic-phased array, (top left) breast coil, and (top right) linear head coil.

Quadrature or circularly polarized types detect signal at 90° apart, which improves the signal-to-noise and efficiency.

The latest coil arrays are described as *multichannel*. Each coil element possesses a separate receiver, and is compatible with parallel imaging techniques to reduce scan time by a factor equal to the number of available channels. A selection of RF coils is shown in Figure 1.13.

> Top Tip! In manual pre-scanning using a multiple-channel array, the nominally displayed receiver may not be the most suitable from which to determine system settings.

Chapter 2
Safety

2.1 INTRODUCTION

A major advantage MRI has over other imaging modalities is its lack of ionizing radiation and inherent safety. Since its introduction into clinical practice in the early 1980s, its use has grown to such an extent that it is estimated that over 20 million scans are carried out worldwide each year. The vast majority of these scans are performed without incident. From my own personal experience, I have volunteered for countless scans, at several different field strengths with no problems (as far as I know!).

Although MRI is an extremely safe form of medical imaging there are three specific interactions between the scanner and the patient that need addressing when quantifying any potential safety hazards. These correspond to the three separate magnetic fields used in the imaging process:

- The static magnetic field produced by the scanner (B_0)
- The time-varying magnetic field produced by the gradient coils (dB/dt)
- The radio-frequency field produced by the imaging coils (B_1)

The following discusses each of these effects in turn together with their appropriate safety limits. In the United Kingdom the Medical and Healthcare Products Regulatory Agency (MHRA) has published guidelines (2002) that do not set exposure limits but intend to draw the attention of users to the limits published by the National Radiological Protection Board (NRPB), and the International Electrotechnical Commission (IEC). The document defines three distinct modes of scanner operation, namely: normal, controlled, and research. Much clearer advice has been proposed by the U.S. Food and Drug Administration (FDA) in 1997 and more recently updated in 2003, which I have used here, and compared alongside the other recommendations.

2.2 STATIC FIELD

Biological Effects

There are no known long-term or irreversible biological effects from exposure to static fields of less than 10 Tesla. This is even more reassuring when you consider that all clinical systems currently operate at no higher than 3.0 Tesla.

There are three forces to consider when examining biological interactions between the human body and the static field of the scanner; these are: translational forces on ferromagnetic objects (the *projectile effect*), torque or turning forces exerted on implants and tissues, and the force induced on moving charged particles. Potentially hazardous effects on human biology involving minute ferromagnetic particles in tissues and moving electrons and ions in cells have been studied and it is well established that these simply could not occur at the field strengths in use.

Some transiently occurring phenomena have been observed, however, at high field. For example, magnetophosphenes (flashing lights in the eyes) have been anecdotally reported at 4.0 Tesla. Other mild sensory effects such as vertigo, nausea, and a metallic taste have also been reported. These have usually been associated with rapid head movements near the entrance of the scanner bore.

In addition there is some alteration in the *T*-wave demonstrated on an electrocardiograph (ECG) trace, which increases at higher field. This is due to the induced electrical potential in moving blood but is of negligible consequence.

Projectiles and Implants

By far the most serious consequence of the static field is the associated projectile risk. The force of attraction is proportional to an object's mass, its susceptibility, the field strength used, and the gradient of this field. Ferromagnetic material (see Chapter 3, What Is Magnetic Susceptibility?) will be accelerated towards the scanner with obvious consequences (Figure 2.1). As a rough rule-of-thumb calculation, a screwdriver can typically reach speeds of around 30 mph near the scanner bore.

The field affects both objects being brought into the scan room and any potential implants within the patient. In particular pacemakers become functionally affected by even small static fields and are an absolute contraindication. The nature and position of implants all have a bearing as to whether they may be scanned. Furthermore, the transition to high field clinical imaging requires careful reassessment: devices tested and

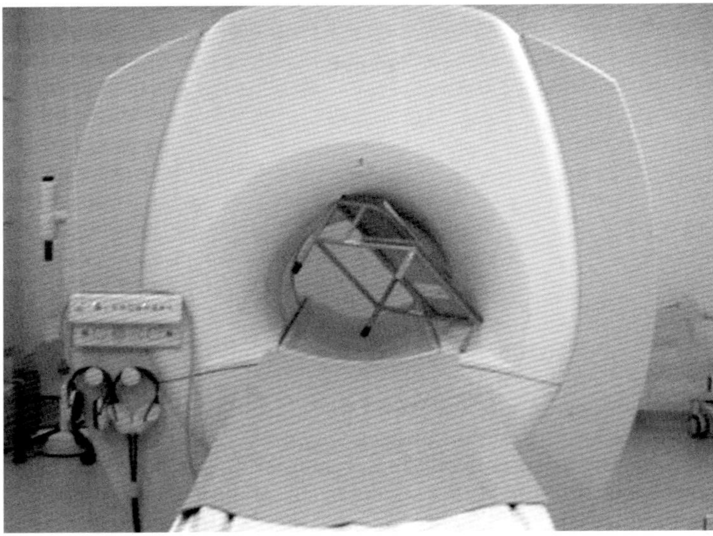

FIGURE 2.1. When things go wrong. . . . Non-MR compatible steps brought into the scan room with obvious consequences.

deemed MR compatible at 1.5 Tesla may no longer be so at higher field strengths.

Of the very few deaths attributed to MRI, only one has been due to projectiles, whereas several more may have been caused by pacemakers or implanted devices.

Safe Operating Limits

The FDA guidelines issued in 1997 stated that the safe exposure to a static magnetic field was limited to 4.0 Tesla. This has now been increased to 8.0 Tesla for most patient populations. The MHRA guidelines consider that use of fields up to 4.0 Tesla constitutes a controlled mode of operation.

The safe fringe field for people with pacemakers (and therefore the proximity limit for members of the general public) is 5 Gauss (equal to 0.5 m*T*).

2.3 TIME-VARYING MAGNETIC FIELD

dB/dt

The gradient coils produce changes in magnetic field over short periods of time, the so-called dB/*dt* effect. With improving technology, gradients have been operating at ever faster switching rates to speed up image acquisition. These rapidly varying fields induce oscillating currents in the human body and have the potential for involuntary stimulation of nerves and muscles. The lowest threshold of patient stimulation is *peripheral nerve stimulation* (PNS). Many studies have been performed on volunteers and demonstrated the onset of PNS at gradient levels of between 60 and 100 T/s. The exact threshold of stimulation is complicated by coil geometry and current waveforms and the longer the pulse duration the lower this threshold becomes. PNS can be used as a subjective indicator that safety thresholds have been reached. Models have shown that cardiac stimulation and ventricular fibrillation occur at much greater thresholds than for PNS with gradient rise times of less than 1 ms, which is far longer than those currently utilized.

Acoustic Noise

The most obvious dB/dt effect the patient will encounter is the loud noise in the scanner bore during the examination. It is a consequence of the force exerted on the gradient coils due to the rapidly varying current within them in the presence of the main field. The frequency of the current is such that the coils vibrate against their surroundings and produce noise at an acoustic level. This noise, which increases with field strength and varies considerably with the type of sequence being used, is sufficient to warrant ear protection for all patients.

High field systems have had to be designed with methods of reducing this noise, most recently incorporating a vacuum-lined bore to attenuate the noise transmitted to the patient. With this technology in place, a modern 3.0 Tesla scanner is not significantly noisier than a 1.5 Telsa system.

Safe Operating Limits

The FDA guidelines state that the gradient levels should not exceed values that produce "severe discomfort or painful nerve stimulation." IEC limits are set at the PNS threshold, and NRPB recommends a limit of $20\,T\,s^{-1}$ for pulses of longer duration than $120\,\mu s$.

In earlier safety publications acoustic noise was not specified. The 1997 and 2003 FDA guidelines indicate that hearing protection should be worn and that peak sound levels of 140 dB should not be exceeded. This corresponds to a "human-ear" weighted value of 99 dBA (also specified by IEC).

2.4 RADIO-FREQUENCY FIELD

Specific Absorption Rate

The concern here is the heating effect and subsequent thermal stress in the human body due to the energy deposited by repetitive RF pulses. The degree of heating is expressed as the specific absorption rate (SAR) in joules per kg of tissue. This value increases with field strength, a fact which is exacerbated by the increased conductivity of the patient at higher field leading to poorer signal penetration prompting the need for higher RF power.

Many studies have been performed in animals and humans over a variety of conditions, varying both the amount of SAR and the duration of the exposure. Changes in heart rate, blood pressure, and body temperature have been monitored and shown to be insignificant.

However, poor positioning of the RF coil cable in combination with a high SAR scan may result in a burn to the patient. This is the most common adverse reaction in MRI but virtually unknown at low field strengths.

Safe Operating Limits

The FDA limits for SAR consist of a whole-body average of 4 W/Kg over a 15 minute period. A correspondingly lower figure of 3 W/Kg is given in the head for any 10 minute period. The threshold increases to 8 and 12 W/Kg for a 5 minute duration in the head/body and extremities, respectively. Equivalent IEC and NRPB criteria are broadly similar but additionally specify a controlled operating mode limit with whole-body temperature rises of no greater than 1°C.

2.5 OTHER ISSUES

Contrast Agents

MR contrast agents are in general far less of a risk than those associated with x-rays and few reports of adverse effects have been noted. By far the most commonly used MR contrast agents are the gadolinium-chelates. Of these Gd-DTPA has been in clinical use the longest, since the late 1980s, and has a proven safety track record. It is currently licensed for doses of up to 0.3 mmol/kg body weight in Europe (0.1 mmol/kg in the United States). Studies have shown very few minor reactions (1 to 4%) typically including nausea, headaches, or a cold sensation at the site of injection. Severe anaphylactic reactions have occurred but these are extremely rare (<0.001%). The effects on the fetus are not certain and only in exceptional circumstances is contrast administered in pregnancy.

Non-gadolinium-based agents have been studied over a relatively shorter period of time but are not known to be any less safe. Particulate agents (e.g., ferumoxides) have a higher incidence of side effects, for example, severe back pain (3%).

A list of MR contrast agents can be found in Appendix II, Section A2.1.

Claustrophobia and Sedation

Although not thought of as a major safety issue, patient anxiety and claustrophobia (specifically the fear of enclosed spaces) may be sufficient in some instances to prevent the completion of the scan. Published figures for the percentage of aborted scans in these situations vary widely from 1 to 20%. Undoubtedly, the type of scan (e.g., use of head coil) and the method of entry (head or feet first) makes a significant difference. Methods to improve patient comfort, not only to alleviate stress but also to minimize movement, include bore lighting, ventilation, and head coil mirrors (see Figure 1.13) to maintain visible contact with staff outside the scanner. For certain scans music may be played through headphones to further relax the patient. Although the number of MR scans being performed continues to rise, modern scanner designs with shorter and wider bores, will help reduce the relative number of failed examinations.

Even with patient-friendly scanners, some adults will refuse to enter the magnet bore. Most of these patients can be scanned after a relatively small (anxiolytic) dose of intravenous benzodiazepine, usually less than 10 mg. Administration of sedation in MR is potentially dangerous and requires adequate monitoring and staff training. Most small children and a few adults will require general anesthetic with the major technical problems that this entails.

> Top Tip! Spend time explaining the procedure to the patients, showing them that both ends of the bore are open. This may be the difference between a successful good quality scan or none at all.

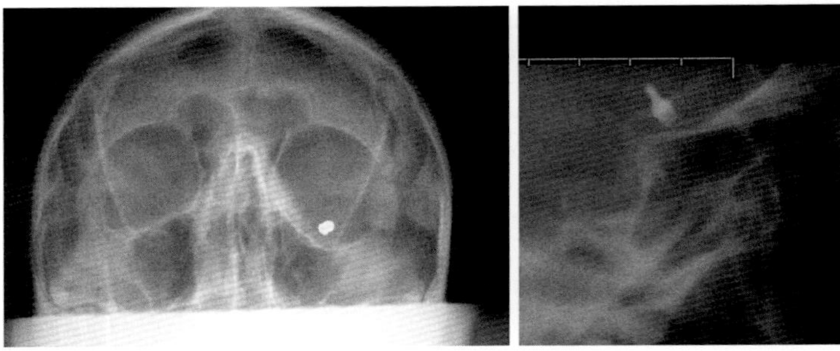

FIGURE 2.2. (left) An orbit x-ray taken as part of patient screening reveals this air-gun pellet. (right) This x-ray, taken to investigate a possible foreign body in the orbit, revealed an aneurysm clip from previous surgery.

Magnet Quench

A quench refers to the sudden loss of the superconductivity of the magnet leading to its nonzero electrical resistance. This in turn produces heat, which causes the cryogens to boil off violently. In the event of this happening, these potentially dangerous gases should be safely vented from the top of the scanner.

2.6 PATIENT SCREENING

Patient screening is the vital first step in any MRI examination. The patient should be asked about any history that may contraindicate the scan. This will include questions concerning previous work with lathes or incidents with metal fragments, with any uncertainty being resolved with an orbit x-ray (Figure 2.2). The presence of any implants (e.g., aneurysm clips) or devices should also be established and removal of all loose metallic objects is mandatory.

Female patients of childbearing age will also be asked whether they could be pregnant. Although there is no firm evidence to suggest any risk, no patients within the first trimester are scanned unless there is a life-threatening reason not to do so. Previous history of adverse reactions to contrast agents should also be noted.

For completeness, an example screening form is provided in the Appendices.

Current Practice at 3.0 Tesla

It is important to emphasize that equipment in regular use at 1.5 Tesla *may not* necessarily be deemed compatible at 3.0 Tesla. At our institution, we have placed additional restrictions regarding the 3.0 Tesla scanner. These include the removal of spectacles (where nonessential for the completion of the scan), and the removal of belt buckles and all items of jewelry (except wedding rings) for head/neck scans. In addition, all clothing (including brassieres but not other underwear) has to be removed for abdomen/pelvic examinations.

Chapter 3
Scan Parameters and Image Artifacts

3.1 SCAN PARAMETERS

Introduction

The signal-to-noise ratio (SNR) is fundamental to the quality of the final image. The signal determines the brightness of each image pixel and is proportional to the RF signal emitted by the tissue. The noise is due to random RF emissions, the main contributor of which is the patient. In this section the effect of changing pulse sequence parameters on SNR, and image quality generally, is discussed. It is always important to remember that any change in the sequence parameters will lead to some trade-off in image quality.

To examine these changes, a "gold standard" T_2-weighted image in the normal brain (shown in Figure 3.1) was acquired with a FSE sequence using the following parameters.

- $TE/TR = 102/3825$ ms.
- 512×384 image matrix, with a 24 cm field of view.
- 5 mm slice thickness with a 1 mm gap.
- 2 signal averages and a bandwidth of 20.8 kHz.

A three-quarter phase field of view (18 cm) was used in the right–left direction (see also Chapter 6, What Is Half-Phase Field of view). In each of Figures 3.2 to 3.5 one particular sequence parameter has been altered to illustrate the effect on image quality.

Signal Averaging

In Figure 3.2 the number of signal averages has been reduced from two to one. Signal averaging works on the principle that the signal is coherent whereas noise is incoherent or random. By recording the signal more than once the effects of the noise can be reduced whereas the signal is constant. The actual improve-

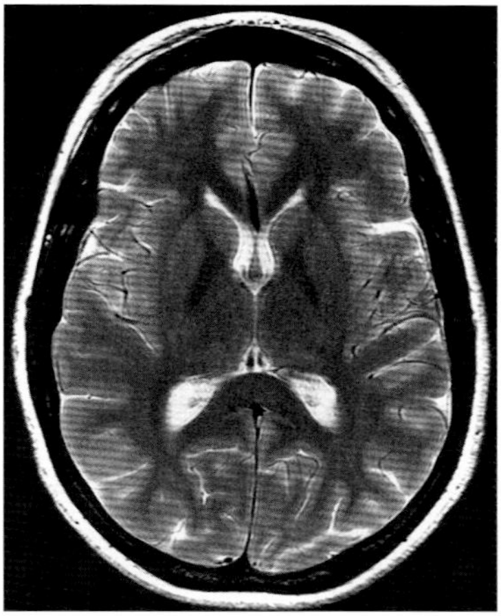

FIGURE 3.1. The gold standard image acquired with sequence parameters as indicated in the text.

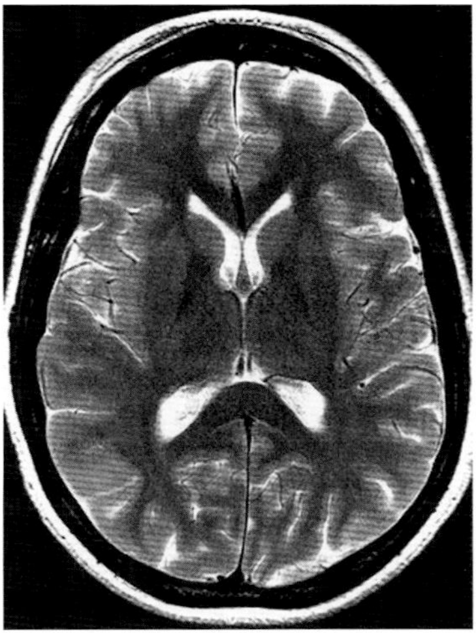

FIGURE 3.2. Image acquired as in Figure 3.1 with the number of signal averages reduced to one.

ment in SNR is a square root of the number of measurements, and in this case SNR is reduced by approximately 30% as can be seen from the image. It should be noted, however, that the image acquisition time is now only half that of the original scan.

Bandwidth

Receiver bandwidth has an inverse square root relationship with SNR. An increase in bandwidth means increasing the range of frequencies at which noise can be encoded, thereby reducing SNR. In Figure 3.3(a) the bandwidth has been reduced to 6 kHz and there is a noticeable improvement in image quality (nearly double). Figure 3.3(b) shows a reduction in SNR owing to the increase in bandwidth (approximately 2.5 times worse).

> Top Tip! If there are too many slices, forcing the scanner into a second acquisition, this can be avoided by extending the receiver bandwidth.

Slice Thickness

SNR is proportional to the amount of spins present and therefore directly related to the slice thickness. Figure 3.4 has been

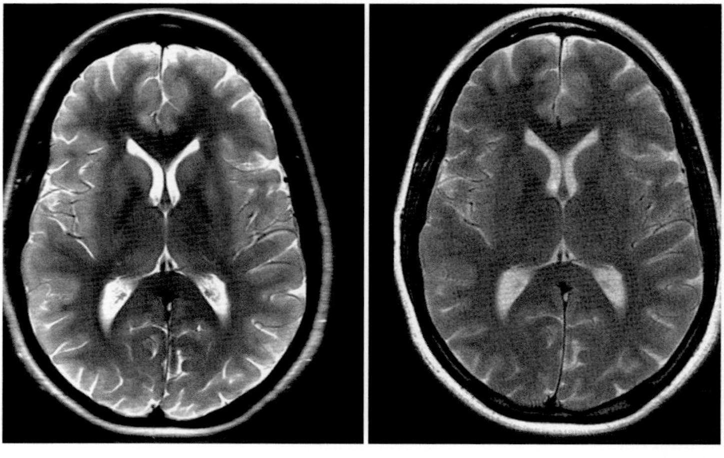

FIGURE 3.3. (left) Bandwidth reduced to ±6 kHz; (right) Bandwidth increased to ±125 kHz.

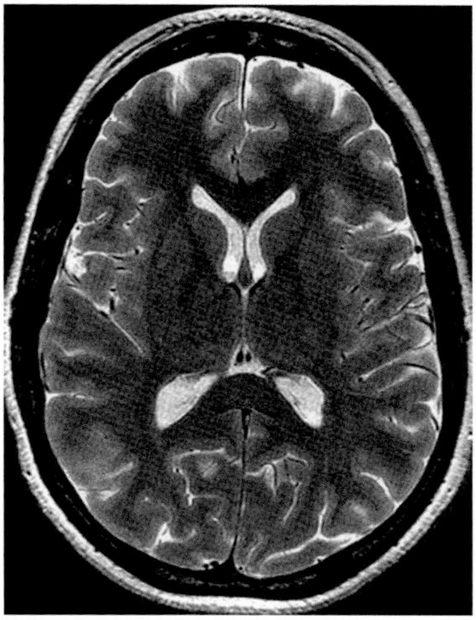

FIGURE 3.4. Slice thickness reduced to 2 mm, resulting in reduced SNR.

acquired with a slice thickness of 2 mm and shows a proportional reduction in SNR (60%). Increasing the slice thickness may result in *partial volume* effects where the signal is an average contribution of different components reducing the contrast of small structures.

Contrast Weighting

The images in Figure 3.5 have been acquired with a longer and shorter echo time producing more and less T_2-weighting, respectively. The CSF in the left image appears bright due to the long T_2 values of fluids.

Factors that influence contrast in the image have a detrimental effect on SNR. For example, longer *TE*s increase T_2-weighting but the signal will be weaker. Similarly, allowing the signal to fully recover (long *TR*) will improve SNR but reduce T_1-weighting.

RF Coil

The choice of RF coil used in signal transmission/reception is crucial. Noise in an image arises from the entire sensitive volume of the coil so it is important to use the smallest possible coil to suit the anatomy being imaged in order to maximize SNR.

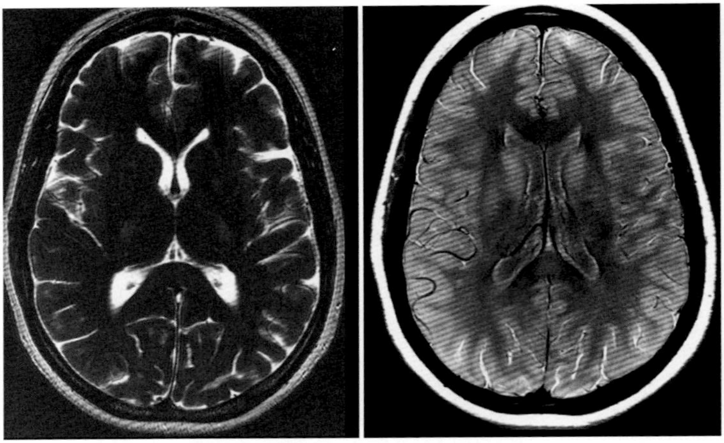

FIGURE 3.5. (left) TE increased to 300 ms to accentuate the T_2-weighting; (right) Low TE to produce more mixed (proton-density) weighting.

B_1 homogeneity is another important feature of the coil. Surface coils will have a poor reception profile leading to a marked signal decrease away from the coil (for example, the spine image in Figure 5.8 and the prostate in Figure 7.3 demonstrate rapid signal drop-off). These inhomogeneities may be sufficiently bad enough to warrant the use of image normalization techniques such as SCIC (see Chapter 7, What Is Intensity Correction?).

Spatial Resolution

The image is subdivided into pixels the dimensions of which are determined by the matrix size and the field of view. Just as slice thickness controls the amount of signal detected, changing the in-plane dimensions will be a trade-off between SNR and spatial resolution. Halving the dimension of the pixels in each direction (by increasing the matrix or reducing the field of view) will reduce the voxel size and SNR by one quarter. In Figure 3.6, the image on the left has been acquired with a 512 × 512 matrix, whereas the image on the right has only a 128 × 128 matrix. The area of each pixel therefore varies from one image to the next by a factor of 8: the image on the left has pixels of 0.22 mm^2 whereas the image on the right has pixels equal to 3.5 mm^2. This results

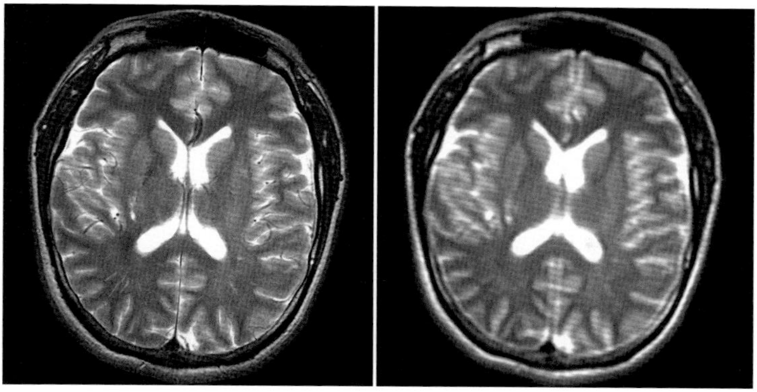

(a) (b)

FIGURE 3.6. Axial brain images with (a) 0.47×0.47 mm in-plane resolution and (b) 1.88×1.88 mm in-plane resolution.

in a dramatic loss of spatial resolution, and image detail such as the vessels seen on the left are simply not visible on the right. Note however, that the image on the right has higher SNR. Generally, resolution should be suited to the anatomy of interest.

3.2 IMAGE ARTIFACTS

An artifact is any property or effect observed in an image that does not appear in the original object. This may range from being a general degradation of image quality and may be easily explainable, to more subtle defects. This section deals with the most common artifacts in MRI. Each case begins with a quick summary of each type: their orientation, related scan parameters, and how they may be minimized, together with a list of other associated names.

Aliasing

- Observed in the phase-encoding direction
- Related to FOV
  - ✓ Swap phase direction or increase FOV
- ➢ AKA: wrap (phase wrap), foldover

Aliasing is more commonly referred to as simply *phase-wrap* as this artifact usually affects only the phase-encoding direction.

Phase-wrap occurs whenever anatomy extends beyond the imaging field of view (FOV). Phase can no longer be unambiguously attributed to each point in the object and results in the offending anatomy being mis-mapped or wrapped into the opposite side of an image. In 3D imaging it will also be present in the third dimension and may be accommodated by maintaining a gap of air or using saturation bands to eliminate any offending signal.

Figure 3.7 demonstrates phase-wrap in an image taken as part of the series of images acquired for Section 3.1. In this case the reduced phase-encoding dimension (18 cm) has been deliberately swapped to run in the anterior-posterior direction. This leads to the wrapping of a small section of the posterior part of the head on top of the anterior part of the image.

Phase-wrap can be avoided by changing the direction of the phase encoding where appropriate or simply increasing the imaging field of view although this results in a reduction of spatial resolution. Most modern scanners provide automatic removal of phase-wrapping as an imaging option (see below).

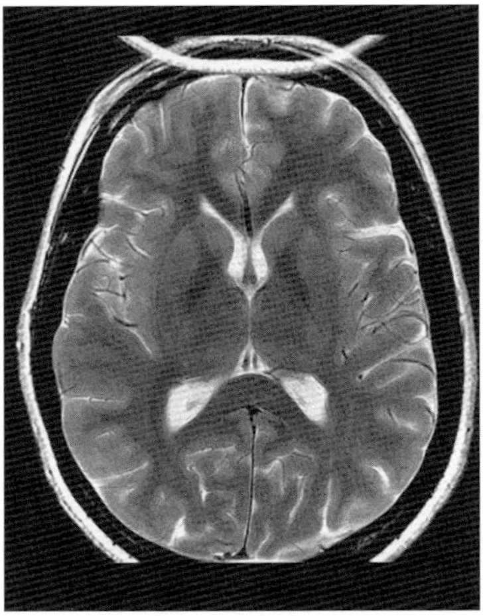

FIGURE 3.7. The smaller phase-encoding dimension has been swapped to run along the anterior–posterior direction resulting in phase-wrap in this image.

Aliasing in the frequency direction is a consequence of the *Nyquist theory*. This states that the signal must be sampled at at least twice the rate of the highest frequency component to be correctly measured. Failure to do this leads to the signal being incorrectly assigned a lower frequency and results in "wrapping" in the frequency direction. However, frequency aliasing is seldom a problem due to the use of high-frequency filters and over-sampling of the signal by the scanner.

❖ What is "No Phase-wrap"?
No phase-wrap (also known as fold-over suppression) is an imaging option available on most scanners. It is used whenever the image prescription is such that wrap is unavoidable, for example, using a small FOV. Basically, the scanner extends the imaging FOV, increases the matrix as necessary to maintain resolution, and may reduce the number of signal averages to limit the increase in scan time. Only the desired FOV is then displayed.

Ringing

- ○ Observed in either direction but often phase-encoding
- ○ Related to matrix dimension
  - ✓ Increase matrix size
- ➢ AKA Gibbs or truncation artifact

Ringing is a consequence of the finite digital sampling of the continuous analogue MR signal. It is evident at high-contrast interfaces where truncation of the Fourier series manifests itself as high signal oscillations (called "Gibbs' overshoot") creating a banding or ringing in the image.

A common place to observe this effect is in the cervical spine as shown in Figure 3.8. In this case, artifactual parallel lines of high signal intensity within the cord can be seen in this T_2-weighted image. The artifact is highlighted in the inset, which shows a section of the cord, and has been magnified and windowed to emphasize the effect.

The artifact is often most prevalent in the phase-encoding direction as this is the matrix dimension, which is often made smallest due to scan time constraints. It may be minimized by increasing the matrix dimension with the penalty of reduced signal-to-noise and extended scan time.

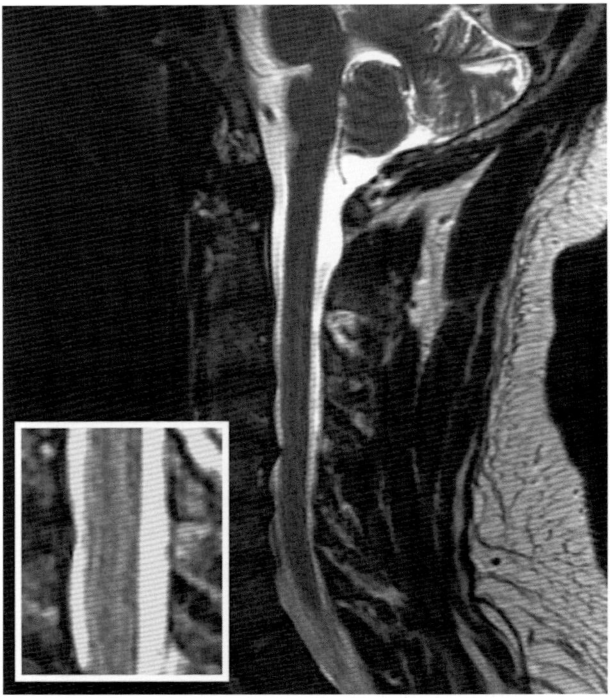

FIGURE 3.8. Artifactual lines of high signal appear in the spinal cord due to ringing (shown in inset).

Ghosting

- ○ Observed in either direction but usually phase-encoding
- ○ Related to scan time
  - ✓ Gating and/or breath-hold for certain periodic motion
- ➢ AKA motion artifact

Ghosting describes the appearance of signal intensity that is above the background noise level of the image. It can occur due to system instability but the most likely cause is patient motion. Depending on the nature of the motion it may be appear as a discrete set of lines, from a periodic source (e.g., cardiac motion) or as a more continuous smear due to nonperiodic motion (e.g., swallowing). It is nearly always observed in the phase direction

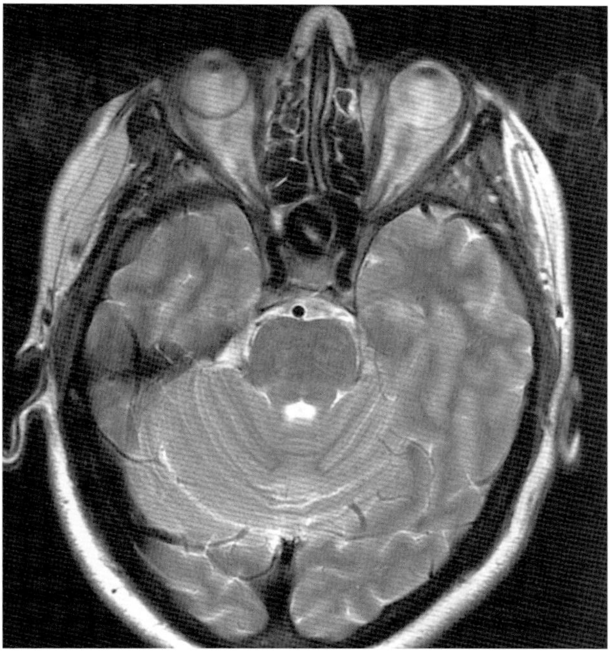

FIGURE 3.9. Ghosting in this image is produced by movement of the eyeballs during the scan.

as the time taken to fully phase-encode an image is long compared to the physiological motion concerned.

In the example in Figure 3.9, movement of the eyeballs during this brain scan has produced marked ghosting in the phase direction (right to left). The propagation of the artifact is along this direction although the motion itself occurs over a small displacement, illustrating the nature of Fourier reconstruction in MRI.

Top Tip! Always ask patients to close their eyes when scanning orbits, as this tends to minimize eye movement.

Ghosting may be reduced in the case of periodic motion by gating the image sequence, ensuring that the phase-encoding steps are acquired at the same time point in the cycle concerned. Both cardiac and respiratory gating is in use although the latter has now been largely replaced by the use of short scan times so that the images are acquired in a single breath-hold (see Sections 7.2 and 7.5 for more on motion compensation).

Nonperiodic motion is harder to overcome and to a large degree relies on patient cooperation and restraint. However, emerging k-space sampling strategies (e.g., PROPELLER) are now being used to good effect.

Artifacts caused by pulsatile blood flow may be reduced by using saturation bands placed outside the imaging slice.

Susceptibility

- Observed in either direction as signal voids/distortions
- Dependent on tissue/material differences
  - ✓ Reduced effect with small voxel size and short *TE*

This artifact occurs at interfaces of materials or tissues with hugely differing magnetic susceptibilities (see Figure 3.10). This is often due to the presence of a foreign body or implant but is also prevalent at air–tissue boundaries, for example, in the orbits. The differing susceptibilities create a local change in the magnetic field, resulting in signal dephasing, which can cause both signal voids and enhancements. Furthermore, frequency differences are superimposed onto the linear imaging gradients and produce geometric distortions.

Susceptibility effects are reduced by using smaller imaging voxels and shorter echo times. In certain instances, they can also be minimized by swapping the phase/frequency directions and using a longer echo train length. However, the artifact becomes worse at high field and is more prominent with gradient-echo sequences due to the T_2* weighting. In certain instances, for example, when using MR-compatible needles, the artifacts demonstrate a prominent dependence on the material orientation in the scanner.

❖ What is Magnetic Susceptibility?
It is a property of matter, which determines how easily it becomes magnetized. Interactions between electrons in the material and an external field cause the field to be either augmented (paramagnetic material, with a positive

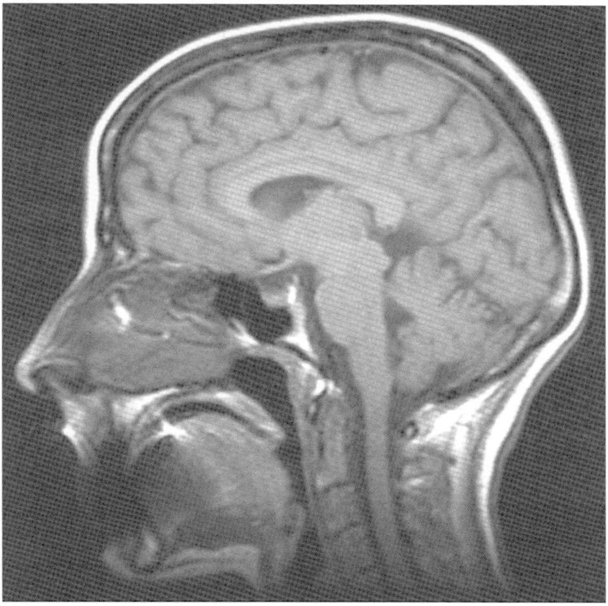

FIGURE 3.10. Susceptibility artifact observed in the mouth of this patient due to dental fillings. It produces signal changes and geometric distortion.

susceptibility) or dispersed (diamagnetic, with a negative susceptibility). Some materials (e.g., iron), described as ferromagnetic, have huge positive susceptibility and become projectiles when brought into the scan room.

Chemical Shift Artifact

- Observed in frequency encoding direction
- Related to bandwidth and frequency matrix
  - ✓ Increase the Hz/pixel ratio
- ➢ AKA Fat-water or black-boundary/relief artifact

This artifact arises due to the frequency difference between the two main components of the signal, namely, water and fat. At 1.5 Tesla the fat resonance is approximately 220 Hz smaller than that of water. The magnitude of the effect is related to the frequency encoding matrix and the receiver bandwidth. Dividing the band-

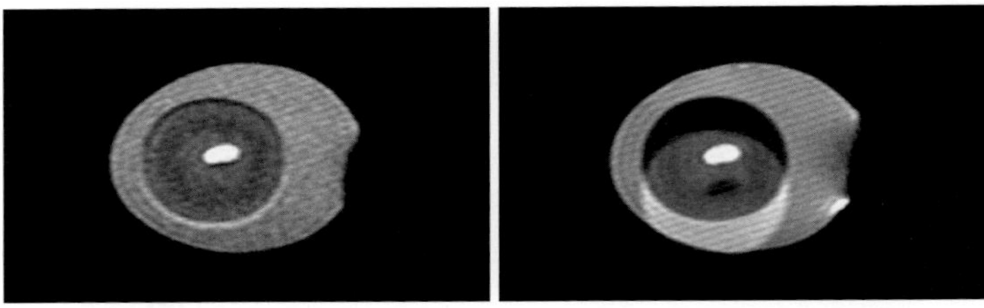

FIGURE 3.11. Images of an egg acquired at two different bandwidths (left) ±32 kHz, and (right) ±3.9 kHz. All other parameters were kept constant.

width by the matrix size determines the spread of frequencies that are available to encode each pixel. If this range is not large enough to encompass the 220 Hz difference, then the fat and water signal, which appears at the same point in the object, will become spatially separated in the final image.

For example, an image with 256 pixels in the frequency direction using a bandwidth of 64 kHz has 250 Hz per pixel (=64,000/256) and there will be no fat–water separation. If the bandwidth is halved, the frequency per pixel is reduced to 125 Hz and fat and water will be separated by nearly two pixels.

The artifact manifests itself as a characteristic signal void and signal increase along opposite sides of the affected tissue due to the spatial misregistration in the frequency direction. An egg provides a great demonstration of this effect. Two images acquired with different receiver bandwidths are shown in Figure 3.11. The image on the left has a light band along the bottom of the yolk and a dark band along the top. At the lower bandwidth (right), the effect is even more pronounced as the fat and water become further displaced.

In vivo the effect is often seen around the kidneys and in the spine, at the junction of vertebral bodies and discs (Figure 3.12).

A related artifact is often termed a chemical shift artifact "of the second kind". It is a consequence of the phase differences between the fat and water signals and is observed in gradient-echo sequences owing to the lack of a 180° refocusing pulse. More specifically it may be observed at certain field-dependant echo times, when the fat and water signals become out of phase leading to signal cancellation and voids in an image. The period is related to the reciprocal of the frequency difference (=1/220) and at certain *TE*s the signals fall alternatively in or out of phase.

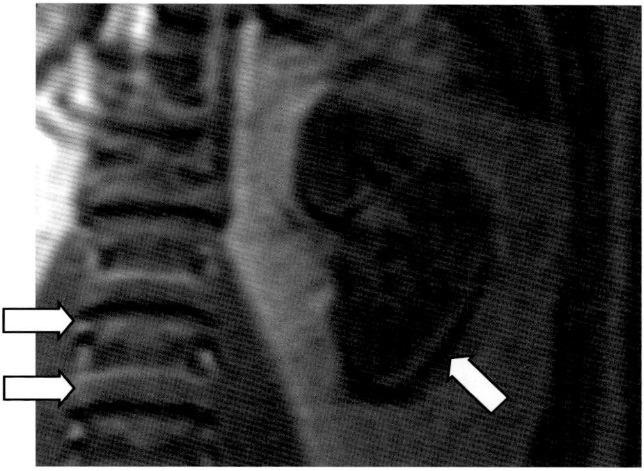

FIGURE 3.12. In vivo example. Here the effect can be seen in the vertebra and around the kidney (frequency direction is top to bottom).

On most MR scanners the user can select the echo time on gradient-echo images to be either in-phase or out-of-phase. In certain sequences (e.g., OOPS), deliberate use of out-of-phase signal cancellation is used to improve tissue visualization (also see Chapter 7).

> Top Tip! Use an out-of-phase *TE* to reduce the fat signal in neck TOF scans.
>
> ❑ *TE* = 2.3/6.9..ms (OUT of phase) and 4.6/9.2..ms (IN) at 1.5 T.
> ❑ *TE* = 1.2/3.5..ms (OUT of phase) and 2.3/4.6..ms (IN) at 3.0 T.

Radio-frequency (RF) Artifact

- ○ Observed perpendicular to frequency encoding direction
- ○ Related to RF interference in the receiver coil
  - ✓ Ensure good RF screening
- ➢ AKA zipper artifact

This artifact is due to interference from either an external RF source (e.g., due to the loss of integrity of the Faraday cage), or from a flickering light bulb within the scan room itself. It may also arise from so-called RF-feedthrough, whereby the receiver picks up signal from the transmitter coil.

It has the characteristic appearance of a stripe or zipper across the image, along the phase-encoding direction and perpendicular to the frequency direction, at the frequency of the interference. It may be a small discrete line or a broader band depending on the source. The example in Figure 3.13 shows the artifact in a shoulder image.

Over-ranging

- ○ Observed throughout image
- ○ Related to signal exceeding the dynamic range of the receiver
  - ✓ Pre-scan usually adjusts so this doesn't happen
- ➢ AKA data clipping, overflow, or halo artifact

This artifact arises as a consequence of incorrectly set receiver gains so that the measured signal causes the amplifier to over-

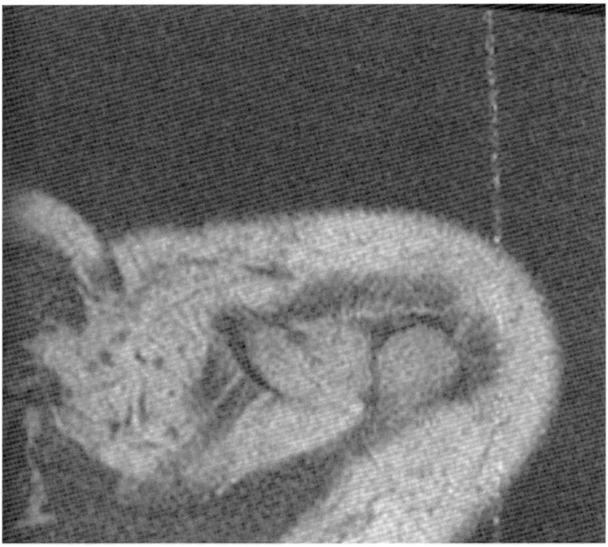

FIGURE 3.13. RF or zipper artifact seen in this shoulder image (frequency direction is left to right).

range. Normally, this is avoided by the pre-scan routine, which sets the transmitter and receiver gains appropriately by playing out the sequence with zero phase-encoding to establish the maximum achievable signal. When this fails, the signal is too large for the analogue-to-digital converter and the data are clipped producing a weird halo of bright signal in the background surrounding a dark center.

The artifact may occur during a dynamic contrast-enhanced scan, when the post-contrast signal exceeds the pre-scan settings. The artifact has been reproduced in Figure 3.14 by simply turning off the extended dynamic range of the scanner and deliberately increasing the receiver gain beyond the value set by the automatic pre-scan routine.

Moire Fringes

- ○ Often observed in 3D gradient-echo imaging
- ○ Related to interference of phase-wrapped signal
  - ✓ Minimize wrap of signal (e.g., suppression or large FOV)
- ➢ AKA zebra artifact

This artifact creates a strange and characteristic banding on the image leading to its alternative name of zebra artifact. It is caused by the interference of aliased signals at different phases. It most commonly occurs in gradient-echo imaging at the periphery of an image volume. The breast image in Figure 3.15 demonstrates Moire fringes (indicated by the arrow).

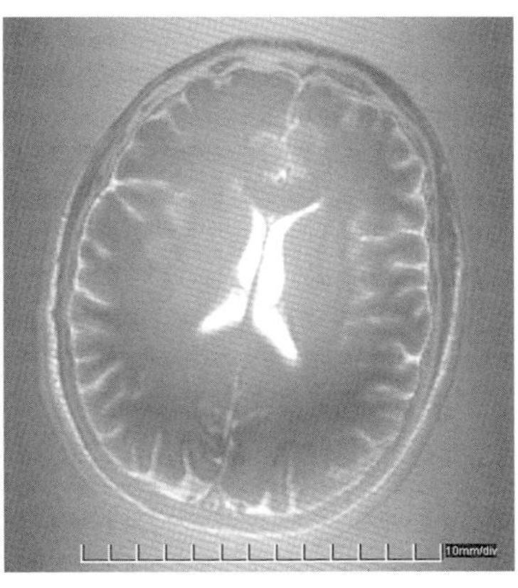

FIGURE 3.14. Example of halo effect caused by over-ranging the RF amplifier.

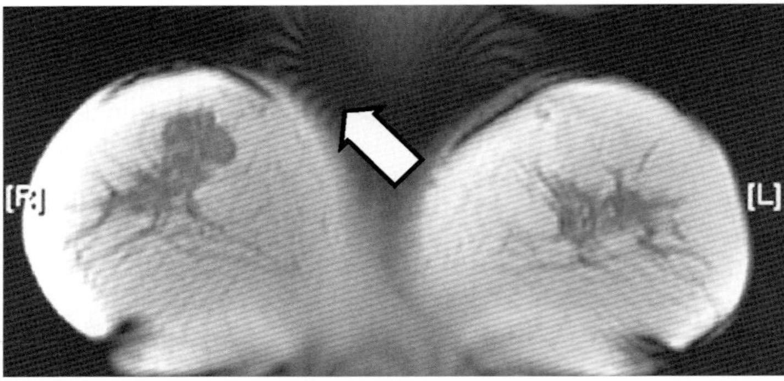

FIGURE 3.15. Example of moire interference fringes observed in this coronal breast image.

Herringbone

- ○ Observed throughout image
- ○ Related to data spike
  - ✓ Reconstruct image without faulty data
- ➢ AKA criss-cross artifact, data corruption error

This artifact is usually a symptom of some transient corruption of raw data. It is often caused by an electrical spike, which Fourier transforms into a sinusoidal function creating a periodic banding across the image. Its characteristic criss-cross pattern gives rise to the name of this artifact. Figure 3.16 shows an example in a breast image. The left half of this image has been windowed differently to show the artifact more prominently.

Standing Wave Artifact

- ○ Higher signal at center of image/general signal variation
- ○ Related to dielectric resonances at high field (3.0 Tesla and above)
  - ✓ Use oil in test objects, dielectric pads in vivo
- ➢ AKA B_1 doming, dielectric, or field-focusing effect

At high field the reduced wavelength of the RF becomes significant in relation to the diameter of the patient and creates resonance effects within the material/tissue being imaged, leading to marked signal variation. In test objects, the high dielectric

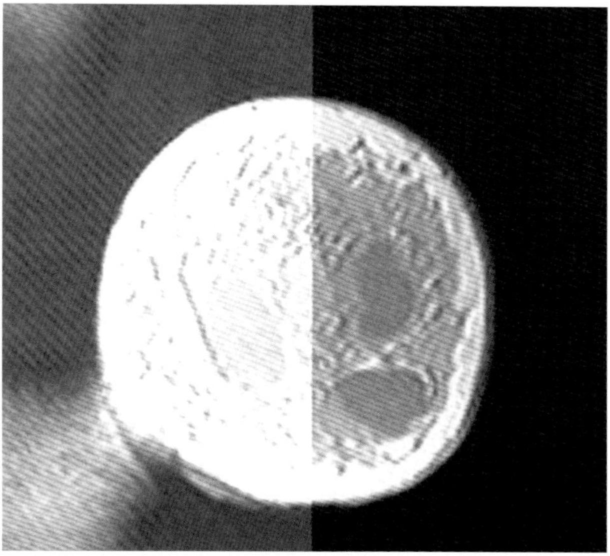

FIGURE 3.16. Herringbone artifact in this breast image (the left half of the image has been windowed differently to emphasize the artifact).

constant (ε) of water makes the problem worse, and the artifact produces so-called *B_1-doming,* where signal at the center is artificially higher than at the edges. It can be overcome by using test objects of smaller diameter or using a material that has a lower ε value (e.g., oil, see Figure 4.2). The high dielectric effect of water may be used advantageously to reduce the signal inhomogeneities seen in vivo (see Figure 7.6, and also Chapter 7, What Is a Dielectric Pad?).

Other Things to Be Aware of. . .

A *central-point artifact* rarely occurs on modern scanners. It is so called as it produces a bright signal spot at the center of the image and is caused by a DC offset in the receiver voltage.

As mentioned earlier, the imperfect nature of slice profiles in 2D imaging leads to the cross-excitation of adjacent slices, which in turn creates dark or saturated signal in the neighboring slice. It is often observed in the lumbar spin at the overlap of differently angled slices (e.g., at L4-5 and L5-S1).

Magic angle effects occur in parallel ligaments or tendons, whose naturally short T_2 values increase when oriented at an angle of approximately 54° to the main field producing a signal increase.

Flow effects may cause artifactual signal enhancements or voids and this is used advantageously in MR angiography. Other MRA-related artifacts include *flow-related aliasing,* when blood flows faster than the *velocity-encoding* threshold causing it to appear black (typically at the center of the vessel). The *venetian blind artifact* is found in multislab TOF techniques. (For more details see Chapter 9.)

System instabilities in the imaging gradients or the main field, will lead to image distortions (also see Section 4.2, Geometric distortion).

Finally, *post-processing* of the image data may introduce its own artifacts. Parameter maps often demonstrate artificial values if there is motion during the acquisition of the data set (an example is given in Chapter 6, What Is Edge Enhancement?). 3D reconstructions will suffer from a steplike appearance (*staircase artifact*) if the original image slices have been acquired too thick.

Chapter 4
Quality Assurance

4.1 THE BASICS

Quality assurance (QA) in MRI has an all-too-often tendency to be overlooked. Unlike imaging modalities involving ionizing radiation, there is no mandatory or legislative requirement to perform quality assessment in MRI. The notion of image quality control varies considerably from medical center to medical center, although it is becoming increasingly recognized as an important aspect of MR practice. By performing a few simple checks on a regular basis, image quality can be verified and any problems highlighted for further investigation. This section gives a brief guide to how QA may be implemented at any MR center.

Fringe Field

The fringe field (also known as *stray field*) is that part of the main magnetic field which extends beyond the imaging field of view. During acceptance testing the field may be measured outside the scan room at certain points using a handheld gaussmeter. The meter should be held at approximately the height of the magnet isocenter, avoiding any screws and the like in the wall. The maximum-recorded value should be checked against the manufacturer's own specifications. This information should be provided on the scanner footprint, a map showing the scanner in situ and the relation of its isofield lines at certain field strengths. The critical safety limit is the *five gauss line* (see Section 2.2, Static Field) and this should be verified as being within a restricted area.

Acoustic Noise

Acoustic noise is not routinely measured, as it requires MR-compatible equipment to be used within the scanner bore. However, with the advent of higher field strengths and the resulting increase in noise levels this may change. Noise should be measured at the isocenter for a variety of imaging sequences and

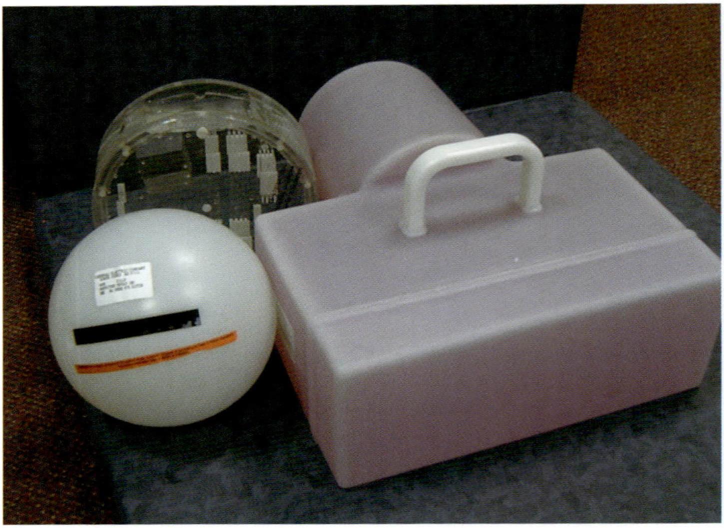

FIGURE 4.1. Selection of MRI test objects (left to right): 1.5 Tesla sphere, Eurospin TO4 (resolution), and a 3.0 Tesla head and neck phantom.

quoted values adjusted for the frequency response of the human ear. The safety aspect of this is discussed in Chapter 2, Acoustic Noise.

Phantoms

Phantoms or test objects are used in the imaging part of QA and can vary considerably depending on their role (Figure 4.1). The simplest test objects tend to be of the uniform flood-fill variety, fluid-filled Perspex spheres and cuboids made to fit specific RF coils. These are used for tests of signal-to-noise ratio, uniformity, and ghosting. In each case they are filled with a solution of a paramagnetic salt (often nickel chloride or similar) to mimic tissue T_1 relaxation times, although the T_2 values are much longer than those in vivo.

For tests such as distortion, slice profile, and resolution, more complicated phantoms are needed. A commonly used set of phantoms is the five Eurospin test objects (referred to as TO1 to TO5). In addition many research sites have their own in-house-built phantoms.

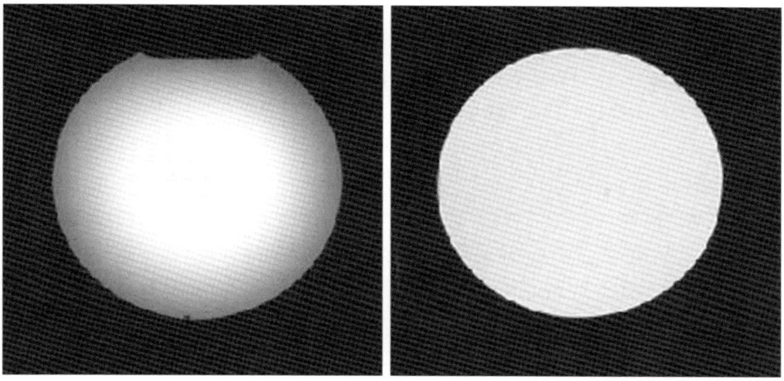

FIGURE 4.2. B_1 doming in a water phantom at 3.0 Tesla (left). The effect is absent when oil is used instead (right).

At higher fields the water must be replaced with oil-based liquids (pink liquid in Figure 4.1) to overcome the dielectric effect, which produces a characteristic signal inhomogeneity called B_1-doming shown in Figure 4.2 (also see Standing Wave Artifact, Chapter 3).

Frequency of QA Checks

Often a manufacturer-specific phantom is provided for daily QA. This is scanned to obtain a quick qualitative assessment of imaging performance, and is usually only carried out for the head coil.

A more rigorous program of tests should be followed shortly after installation of a new scanner and on an annual basis thereafter or whenever there is potential for changes in performance, for example, following a system upgrade. The tests should cover as much of the following measurements as possible using a variety of RF coils (or at the very least the head and body coil) but will depend on the availability of phantoms at each site.

4.2 MEASUREMENTS AND ANALYSIS

The following imaging parameters are usually measured as part of quality assurance of the MRI system. Usually a simple spin-echo sequence is sufficient to carry out the majority of these tests (e.g., using TE/TR = 30/500–1000 ms, 256 × 256 matrix, 5 mm slice). If tests are repeated at a subsequent time, the imaging protocol must remain constant to allow a comparison to be made. Some scanners apply default raw data filters, which should be turned off where possible, as these will affect the measurements taken. It may also be pertinent to record pre-scan settings such as center frequency and transmitter/receiver gains to assess any temporal drift in these values.

> Top Tip! For liquid phantoms, allow time to settle once inside the scanner as fluid motion will give erroneous results.

Signal-to-noise Ratio (SNR)

SNR is the most sensitive test for monitoring system performance but does not specifically indicate the cause of any problems. Rather, it is a useful baseline measure against which future tests may be checked. It is measured using a flood-fill phantom and there are several methods of obtaining SNR. It may be determined from the ratio of the mean to standard deviation (SD) of signal in a region-of-interest (ROI) placed within the phantom acquired over a number of repeat acquisitions. A simpler alternative is to use a single image and record the mean ROI signal and divide this by the SD taken in a background (noise) ROI, away from any ghosting. A third method involves the subtraction of two separate but otherwise identical images, with the SD value taken from the subtracted image at the same position as the phantom ROI. By using appropriate factors in the last two methods, (1) $\sqrt{2-\pi/2}$ to account for noise distribution, and (2) $\sqrt{2}$ for the use of subtracted signal, all three methods should give the same answer.

There is no ideal value for SNR and comparisons among different RF coils is difficult, as it will depend on the filling and quality factors of the coils.

Ghosting

Ghosting (in terms of QA) is present due to system instabilities and may also be measured from the above (SNR) image. The ghost-to-signal ratio (GSR) is recorded using the mean signal in the phantom and the mean ghost signal in a ROI taken within the background along the phase-encoding direction (however, ghosts caused by receiver quadrature problems may appear in a different position). A maximum GSR value should be reported, and typically this should be less than 1% for conventional images rising to 5% for ultrafast gradient-echo sequences (e.g., EPI).

Uniformity

This is a measure of the signal homogeneity. Among the many contributing factors to this, the B_1 sensitivity of the RF coil is the main source. Measurements may again be made from the above images. A line profile of pixel intensity (usually an average of several profiles to reduce data noise) is taken through the center of the image in both directions. This provides a visible check of uniformity; ideally the intensity profile should be flat across the phantom. If a sphere rather than a cylinder is used for this test, the edges of the phantom should be avoided.

A quantitative measure may be obtained from the percentage of pixels with a signal value, which is within 10% of the most commonly occurring pixel intensity at the image center (this is the *fractional uniformity*).

An alternative approach involves measuring the mean and SD from an ROI within the phantom and expressing the *percentage uniformity* as:

$$100 \times (1 - \text{SD/mean}).$$

In both cases values of 100% indicate a perfectly uniform image.

Spatial Resolution

This is assessed using a test object comprised of a set of bar patterns consisting of parallel plates of various thickness and separation distances (Eurospin TO4 or similar). A single pixel profile taken perpendicularly across the bars gives a visible indication as to whether the nominal resolution has been achieved. The resolution may be tested in both directions for phase and frequency encoding. This will involve repeating the image with the encoding directions swapped and again with the phantom rotated 90° to test the orthogonal gradient.

Example data are shown in Figure 4.3 (left). In this case a line profile has been taken across three different sets of plates with thickness/separation equal to 0.5 mm, 2.0 mm, and 1.0 mm (from left to right). The modulation of the peaks and troughs (indicated by arrows) is acceptable if this is 50% or greater. The nominal in-plane resolution of the image in this example was 0.7 mm and as expected the second pattern is completely resolved, whereas the first is not. The third set, which should also

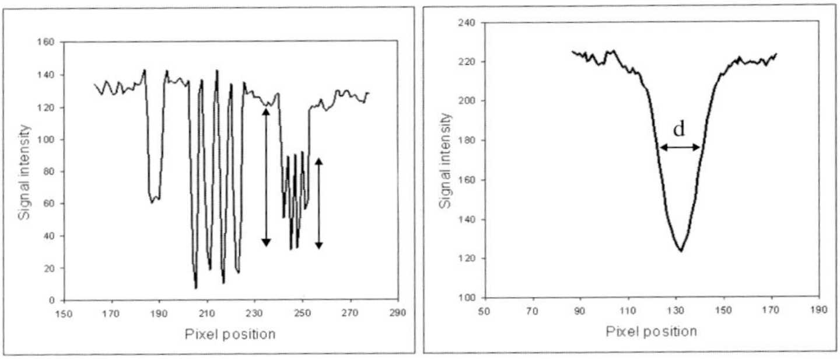

FIGURE 4.3. Example QA data for spatial resolution (left) and slice profile (right) tests.

be resolved, is more borderline. The success of this test relies upon good alignment of the phantom. A more complicated method involves determining the modulation transfer function from a pixel profile taken across the edge of a block.

SLICE PROFILE

A phantom containing a thin angled plate is required for this test (Eurospin TO2 or similar). Imaging should be acquired so that the plate is angled through the image slice. A line profile is taken along the plate to reveal a signal trough (as shown in Figure 4.3, right). The distance across this trough (*d*), recorded at the full width at maximum height (FWHM), is related to the slice thickness by

$$\text{Slice thickness} = d \times \tan\alpha,$$

where α is the angle of the plate. In TO2, a pair of opposite angled plates is incorporated and two measurements may be taken to correct for errors in misalignment of the phantom. Measurements should be taken at different values of slice thickness (e.g., 3 and 5 mm) and results should be within ±10% of actual values, although the method works less well when the slice thickness approaches the dimension of the plate.

Geometric Distortion

This term covers both *linearity* (change in object size and dimension) and *distortion* (displacement of points within an image). The main causes of geometric distortion are problems with the linearity of the gradients and homogeneity of the main field. This is an essential measurement if MRI is to be used for registration with other imaging modalities (e.g., CT for radiotherapy planning). Essentially a phantom comprising plates or rods of known distances over a reasonably large volume (20–40 cm) should be used. These distances are then compared to measurements recorded in the image. Usually several measurements are taken at different locations and the mean and SD are recorded.

Contrast and Relaxation Time Accuracy

A phantom containing objects with a varying range of relaxation times should be used in this case. The *contrast factor* may be measured for different imaging sequences, which is determined by the difference between the highest and lowest signals, divided by the summation of these two signals.

If the relaxation times of the materials have been previously determined (e.g., Eurospin TO5) the accuracy and precision of relaxation time measurement may also be assessed although this depends on the availability of image-processing software.

Signal Stability

This is a particularly important QA measurement for centers implementing functional MRI. A flood-fill phantom should be imaged repeatedly and acquired with the same imaging protocol as that used in a clinical examination (e.g., single-shot EPI or similar, over several minutes). Generally, for gradient-intensive sequences, it is a good idea to "warm up" the scanner by acquiring these data twice and analyzing the repeat measurement. The percentage of signal variation should be recorded and ideally this should vary less than ±0.5% (at 1.5 Tesla) from the baseline value and there should be no significant trend over the time course.

Part II

The remaining chapters of the book are organized into anatomical sections. Relevant techniques are described in detail where they are first introduced, although some of these may equally apply in subsequent sections. In each case there is a brief appraisal of imaging protocols and example sequences are given (definitions can be found in Appendix I). The sequences are included only as a guide and significant variations or alternatives may also be in regular use.

Chapter 5

Brain and Spine

5.1 BRAIN—INTRODUCTION

Since the early 1980s, MRI has been shown to be the most sensitive technique for the vast majority of intracranial disease. MRI is poor for demonstrating fractures in dense cortical bone, and may be difficult in hyperacute hemorrhage and subarachnoid bleeding. For these reasons, CT remains the first investigation for cerebral trauma and suspected intracranial bleeding. Diffusion-weighted imaging is capable of diagnosing acute stroke as soon as the patient presents in hospital. However, these patients are often very sick and CT again remains the primary investigation.

MRI can provide important pre-surgical information in the investigation of brain tumors, that is not apparent with CT, and is the preferred investigation, but is not always obligatory. The benefits are particularly apparent in the temporal lobes and posterior fossa where CT suffers from beam-hardening artifacts. MRI allows the assessment of invasion of venous sinuses by meningioma, the assessment of optimal sites for biopsy in malignant tumors, and monitoring of the response to treatment. It is also the appropriate test for all suspected pituitary disease and in the screening of patients with sensory neural hearing loss.

MRI is very sensitive to disease of the cerebral white matter and is the only sensible imaging test for MS. As long as contrast is used, it is sensitive to diseases involving the pial meninges, which could be otherwise easily missed.

Ideally, MRI would be used for all patients with epilepsy, but certainly for those with focal epilepsy, such as temporal lobe epilepsy (TLE). Its lack of ionizing radiation has specific advantages in children, which usually justifies the need for sedation.

Role of MRI

✓ Ischemia/infarction
✓ Tumor assessment/response to treatment

✓ Multiple sclerosis
✓ Temporal lobe epilepsy

5.2 CONVENTIONAL TECHNIQUES

Protocols

- *Axial T_2–W FLAIR.* The vast majority of intracranial lesions exhibit long T_2 values. FLAIR is a similar sequence to STIR (see Chapter 1) but in this case it uses a longer inversion time (approximately 2200 ms) to suppress CSF and increase conspicuity of the lesion. The axial plane is useful as it is comparable to CT.

*Example sequence: TE/TR/TI = 148 /9200 ms /2200 ms
FOV = 22–25 cm, Slice thickness/gap = 5/1 mm*

- *Sagittal T_2–W FSE.* This plane is excellent for cerebellum, brain stem, corpus callosum, and the pituitary gland.

*Example sequence: TE/TR = 100 ms/5 s,
Slice thickness/gap = 4/1 mm.*

- *Gradient-echo Imaging.* This is used in cases of trauma or where hemorrhage is suspected. The iron content causes dephasing and signal loss due to susceptibility effects on T_2*–W sequence (see Figure 5.1).

Example sequence: FGRE with TE/TR/flip = 20/800 ms/30°.

- *Post-contrast.* This is for intracranial lesions. Administer contrast and then acquire single (static) post-contrast acquisition (dynamic scans are not usually performed).

Example sequence: any standard T_1-weighted sequence.

- *Stroke protocol.* This is the axial T_2–W as above plus diffusion-weighted sequence (see below and Figure 5.2). In addition use an appropriate MRA protocol, for example, TOF in circle of Willis plus CE-MRA of carotids (see MR Angiography Section and Figure 9.3).

Example sequence: DWI spin-echo EPI with b = 1000 s mm^{-2}.

- *Temporal lobe epilepsy.* This is used for investigating hippocampal sclerosis. Use axial T_2–W and Coronal T_1–W

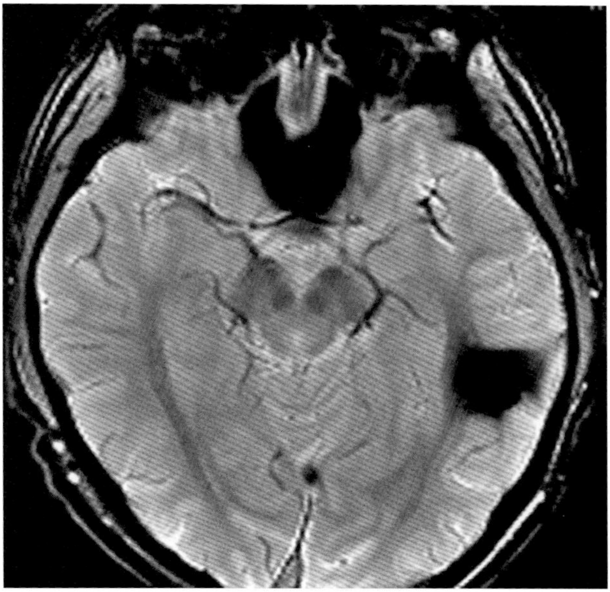

FIGURE 5.1. T_2*-weighted image demonstrates the presence of a hemorrhage.

sequences. Examine loss of internal architecture and signal changes. T_2 mapping may be used to demonstrate elevation of values in effected area.

Example sequence: axial T_2–W FSE, TE/TR = 105/3820 ms. Coronal T_1–W SE, TE/TR = 10/480 ms.

- *Pituitary.* Use coronal T_1–*W* and T_2–*W* with a smaller field of view and thin slices for increased resolution.

Example sequence: Use a 20 cm FOV and 2 mm slice thickness.

- *IAMS/acoustic neuromas.* Use 3D volume to utilize thin sections with increased SNR, for good sagittal reconstructions through each internal ear.

Example sequence: T_1-weighted FSPGR TE/TR/flip = short/ 6.9 ms/30°, Slice thickness = 0.8 mm.

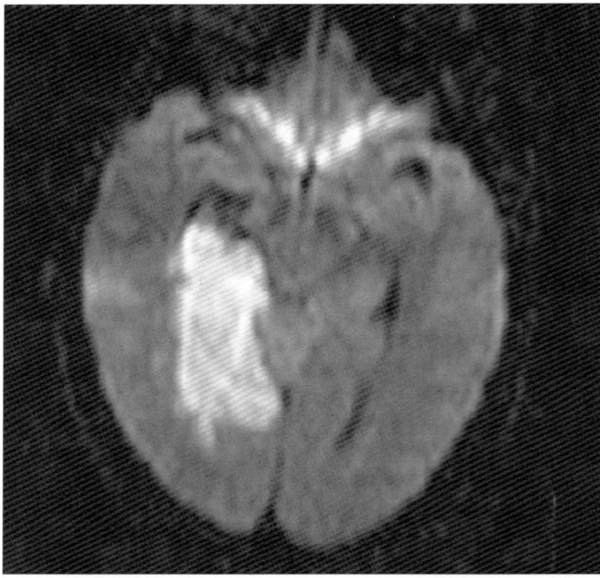

FIGURE 5.2. Diffusion-weighted EPI image with b = 1000 s/mm^2 in a patient following a stroke. The ischemic region is clearly visible as the high signal.

RF Coils

A dedicated head coil is used, typically an optimized birdcage design operating as a transceiver. This type of coil performs best in the axial plane. Early single (linear) channel types are largely being replaced by multielement (usually eight) coils, which improve SNR and can be used for parallel imaging (see What Is Parallel Imaging? in Chapter 1).

Combined head and neck coils are also available for large field-of-view neurovascular work. In addition, specialized surface coils may be used for orbits, which permit greater resolution due to the improved SNR offered by small coils.

Diffusion-weighted Imaging

Diffusion-weighted imaging (DWI) is used in suspected infarction. Cell swelling in the area of ischemia causes a local decrease in diffusion, which appears as an area of hyperintensity on DWI.

The most common method is the PGSE or pulse gradient spin-echo sequence (also known as Stejskal–Tanner). Two strong gradients of opposite polarity are applied with a short interval in between. Any stationary spins are equally dephased and rephased by the action of these gradients. However, spins that move between the two gradients experience a different field at the time of the second application and do not fully recover their phase, leading to signal attenuation. By utilizing strong enough gradients, the sequence is sensitive to microscopic motion such as the diffusion of water. This sensitivity is related to the gradient strength and timings, collectively expressed by the *b*-value.

Examples

Figure 5.1 demonstrates the use of gradient-echo sequences in cases of trauma or where hemorrhage is suspected. The iron content of the hemorrhage produces susceptibility effects leading to signal loss.

Figure 5.2 shows a DWI in a stroke patient obtained with a *b*-value equal to $1000\,s/mm^2$. The reduced diffusion in the ischemic region is exhibited as a region of hyperintensity. Changes on DWI are present within 1 hour compared to 6–12 hours with conventional imaging.

Sometimes, DWI is combined with perfusion-weighted imaging (PWI) to help discriminate viable tissue (see What is PWI?, below). The mismatch between PWI and the DWI can determine whether further treatment (e.g., thrombolysis) is appropriate. PWI is also used to assess the vascularity of tumors.

❖ What is Perfusion-weighted Imaging (PWI)?
PWI refers to imaging that reflects microscopic blood flow. Usually dynamic contrast enhancement is used in conjunction with T_2*–*W* imaging. A signal drop is observed due to the susceptibility effects during the rapid passage of contrast through the capillary bed and this may be quantified to determine cerebral blood flow and volume.

Figure 5.3 shows how contrast enhancement has been used to demonstrate two metastatic tumors. This T_1-weighted image demonstrates two foci of hyperintensity due to the uptake caused by the increased tumor neovascularity.

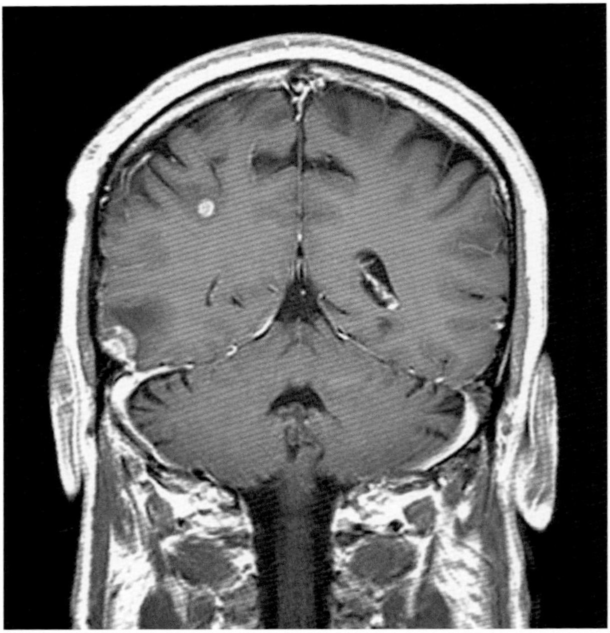

FIGURE 5.3. This contrast-enhanced coronal image demonstrates two metastatic tumors with surrounding edema.

5.3 ADVANCED APPLICATIONS

MR Spectroscopic Imaging (MRSI)

MR spectroscopy permits metabolic information to be investigated by recording chemical shift (see Chapter 1). Multiple voxel techniques are particularly useful in the brain in order to examine heterogeneity within tumors and collectively they may be referred to as MRSI or *chemical shift imaging*. MRSI may be used in a variety of pathologies but by far the most common application is in the investigation of tumor classification and extent. Choice of protocol is influenced by the sequence used: in PRESS, at TE = 135 ms the lactate peaks become inverted and become more easily distinguished from lipids. Shorter echo times produce good SNR but a more prominent lipid signal.

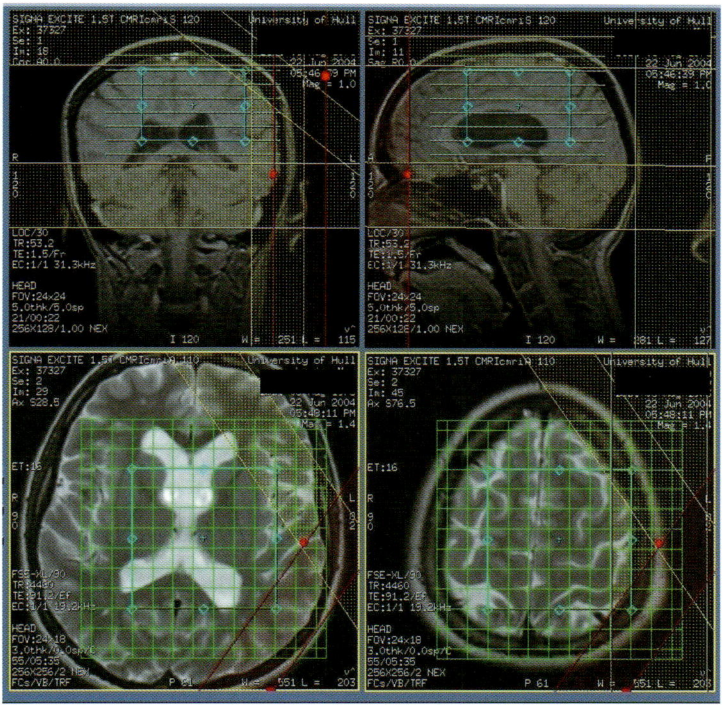

FIGURE 5.4. Graphical prescription of the MRS volume of interest.

Figure 5.4 demonstrates a typical scanner console display during the prescription of a MRSI examination. The spectroscopic volume of interest is displayed in three dimensions (in blue) together with a grid to indicate the locations of the multiple voxels (green). The user may also position saturation bands (red and yellow) to reduce signal contamination from outside the volume.

> Top Tip! Acceptable shimming in 3D MRSI should produce a water peak with a linewidth of 10–15 Hz. A corresponding value for a single voxel exam should be around 7 Hz.

In the brain the metabolites of interest are choline (3.2 ppm), creatine (3.0 ppm), N-acetyl aspartate (NAA, 2.0 ppm), and to a lesser extent lactate (1.3 ppm). NAA is present in normal tissue but reduced in tumors, whereas elevation of choline is indicative of high cell membrane turnover typical in tumor growth. The ratio of choline to NAA is therefore thought to be a useful marker of disease and MRSI can potentially demonstrate the presence of a tumor before changes are seen in conventional imaging.

MRSI data may be displayed as metabolite maps using proprietary software (e.g., GE's Functool). This involves integration of peak areas over a specific chemical shift range and displaying these values in a color scale overlaying the images. Choline and/or NAA are often used but choline-to-creatine has also been used to distinguish recurrence from radionecrosis.

Figure 5.5(a) shows a T_2-weighted image in a patient with a tumor (left). The MRSI grid is positioned over the hyperintensity and the choline–NAA ratios determined in each voxel, with abnormal levels being displayed as varying gray levels (right). In (b) spectra from three voxels have been selected to illustrate normal NAA levels (bottom left) in uninvolved tissue, very abnormal NAA and choline levels (bottom right), and less abnormal levels (top right). Of interest is the discrepancy between the image and MRSI tumor volume.

Example sequences: STEAM single voxel 1 cm^3 using TE/TR = 20–30/2000 ms.

3D MRSI using PRESS with 8 × 8 × 8 (1 cm^3) voxels, with TE/TR = 35/1000 ms (8 min 32 s acquisition time).

Quantitative Diffusion: ADC and DTI

If images with different b-values are acquired, a parameter map of the *apparent diffusion coefficient* or ADC can be determined. This overcomes "T_2 shine-through", or the appearance of high DWI signal in areas of long T_2. Usually, a $b = 0$ image (no diffusion gradient) and one other (in the range, $b = 700–1000\,\text{s/mm}^2$) is used. ADC measurement has been used both in stroke and tumor studies.

For a full three-dimensional characterization the diffusion tensor needs to be determined. This requires at least 6 different b-value images but as many as 55 can be used. *Diffusion tensor imaging* (DTI) is used in the brain to map the white-matter fiber tracts, which restrict diffusion along certain directions. DTI provides rotationally invariant measures such as fractional anisotropy (FA) and diffusion orientation. Tracking algorithms

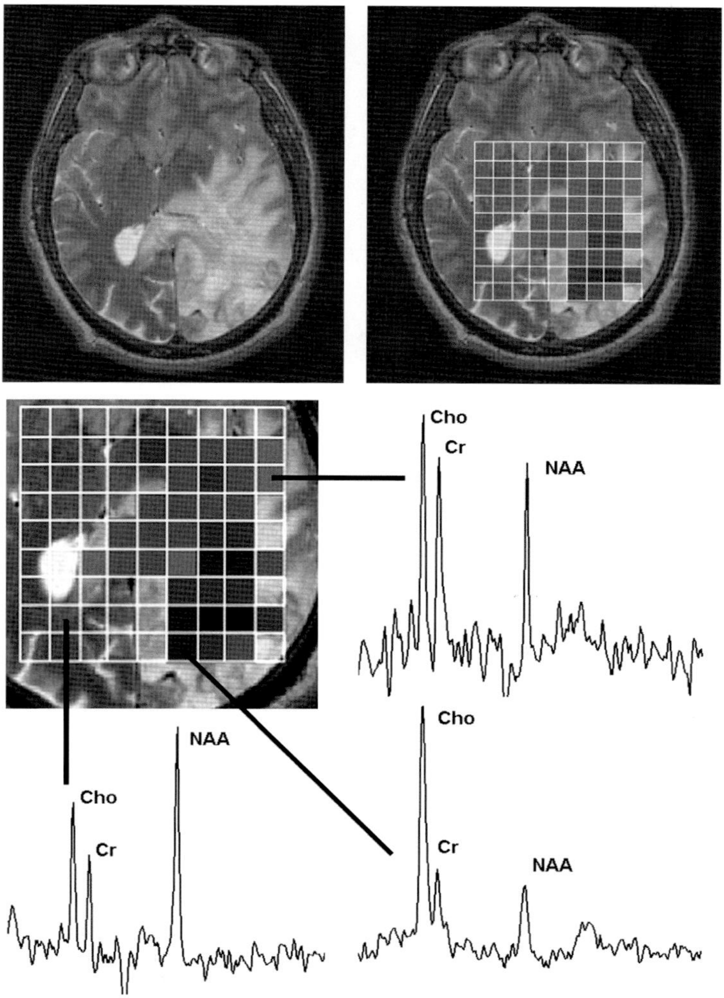

FIGURE 5.5. (a) Example of metabolite mapping in a brain tumor (b). Individual spectra from three voxels of varying NAA:choline ratio are illustrated. (Metabolite maps produced by SIRAMAS software, courtesy of Roberto Garcia-Alvarez.)

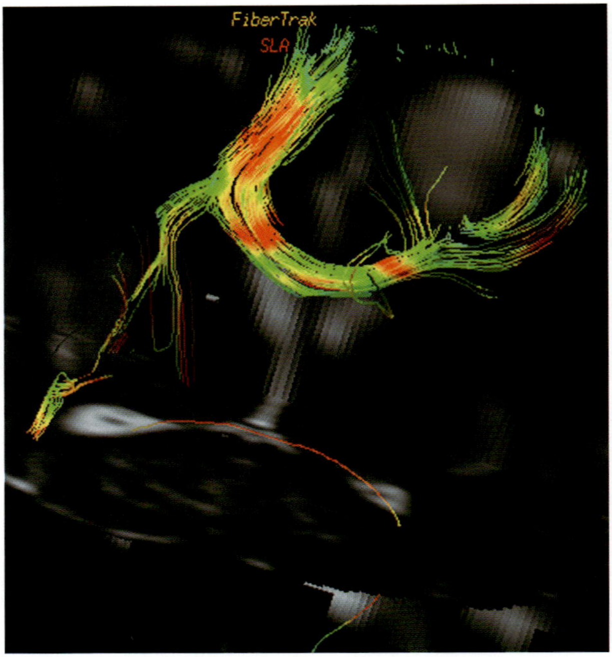

FIGURE 5.6. Fiber tracking in a brain tumor. The fibers have been displaced and can be seen to deviate around this tumor (top right).

can then be used to visualize the fiber trajectories and this is useful in pre-surgical planning. An example is given in Figure 5.6, where the fibers (color coded by FA values) can be seen to deviate around this glioma.

Functional MRI (fMRI)

fMRI permits the noninvasive study of brain function using BOLD (Blood Oxygen Level Dependent) contrast. The technique relies on the hemodynamic response to brain activation to indirectly monitor brain function. Images are repeatedly acquired throughout the brain, during which time the patient is subjected to a task or stimulus interspersed with periods of rest. For example, by prompting the patient to move the fingers of his right hand, activation in the left primary motor cortex will be exhibited. BOLD monitors the change of susceptibility as oxygen flow increases disproportionately in metabolic response to activation. The consequent decrease in paramagnetic deoxyhemoglobin produces a tiny increase in signal intensity on T_2*-weighted images. Using appropriate software, the images are interrogated on a pixel-by-pixel basis and pixels, which correlate significantly with the stimulus pattern, are highlighted in color. These pixels may be overlaid onto a second set of greyscale anatomical images acquired at much greater spatial resolution. Advanced processing corrects for distortion and motion and registers the data to standard Talairach co-ordinates.

> Top Tip! Improve standardization of fMRI in the motor/sensory cortex by acquiring oblique axial scans parallel to the AC–PC line.

Current clinical interest in fMRI revolves around its ability to highlight functioning cortex in patients with intracranial tumors prior to treatment (surgery and radiotherapy) in order to avoid damage to this region.

The technique is also being used as a noninvasive alternative to the WADA test for language lateralization with promising results.

Figure 5.7 shows an example of fMRI being performed to examine the sensory cortex of a patient with a brain tumor. In this case the patient's right hand was stroked during the periods of stimulus to elicit a response in the left sensory cortex, near the location of the tumor.

Example sequence: gradient-echo EPI with TE/TR/flip = 30 ms/3000 ms/90°, typically 20–30 s periods of rest/task repeated three or four times.

5.4 SPINE—INTRODUCTION

MRI is very sensitive to all forms of spinal disease other than fractures. It is the only technique that permits direct imaging of disease involving the spinal cord and is now used as the primary test in almost all spinal patients, and has virtually replaced myelography. Nevertheless, imaging of the cervical and thoracic regions remains one of the most technically challenging areas for MRI, due to the small size of important structures, susceptibility, and flow-related artifacts. Satisfactory results are dependent

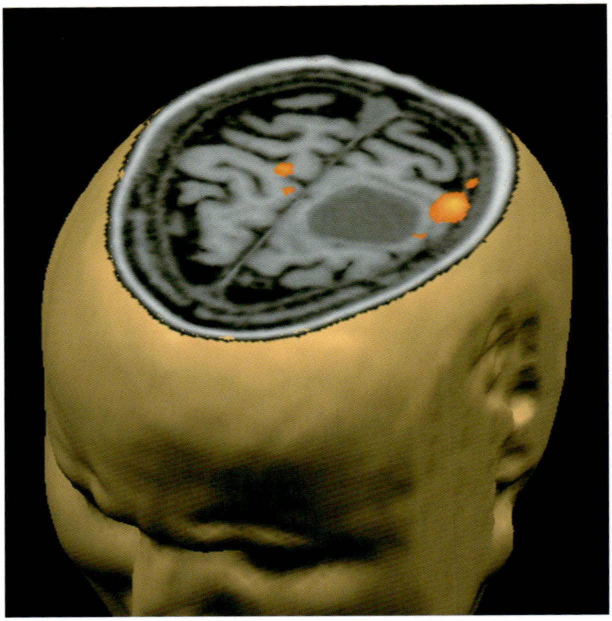

FIGURE 5.7. fMRI study of the sensory cortex in a patient with a tumor.

on high-quality equipment and careful attention to sequence parameters.

Role of MRI

✓ Whole spine: metastatic disease (spinal cord compression), infection, leptomeningeal disease
✓ C Spine: trauma, spinal stenosis, prolapsed intervertebral disc (PID)
✓ T Spine: trauma, spinal stenosis, multiple sclerosis, transverse myelitis, PID
✓ L Spine: Lower back pain, sciatica, and the like, PID

5.5 CONVENTIONAL TECHNIQUES

Protocols

- *Sagittal T_2–W.* T_2-weighting demonstrates cord edema, hemorrhage, and ligament disruption. Use superior/inferior saturation bands to reduce artifacts from venous/arterial flow.

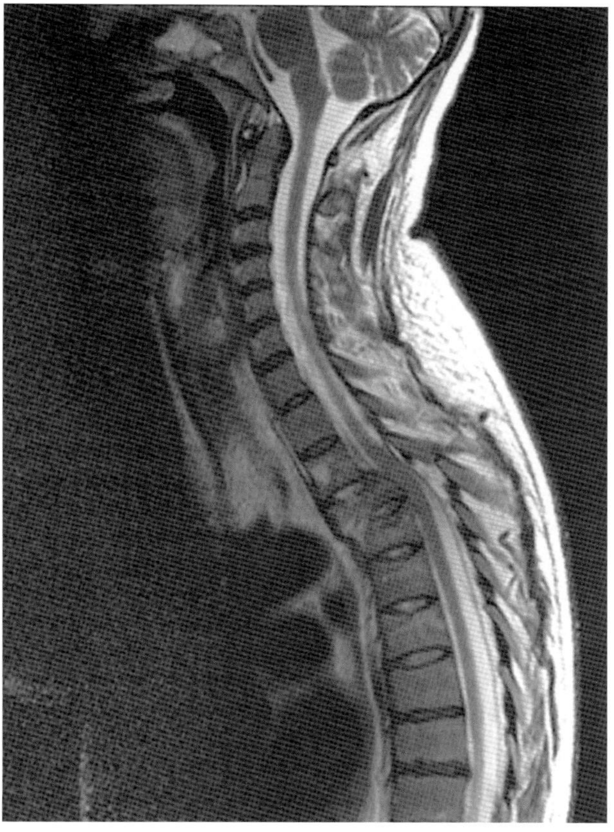

FIGURE 5.8. Sagittal T_2-weighted C-spine image demonstrating trauma.

Example sequence: FSE TE/TR = 83/4200 ms.

- *Sagittal T_1–W.* T_1-weighting demonstrates hemorrhage, bone metastases, and general anatomy.
- *Sagittal STIR.* This is used for cord abnormalities, bone metastases.
- *Axial 3D gradient-echo.* This acquired parallel to the relevant vertebral end plates. For thoracic and lumbar spine, separately angled segments need to be prescribed.

Example sequence: TE/TR/flip = 4/8 ms/45°.
Use 1.5 mm slice thickness.

> Top Tip! Cardiac gating may be used to further reduce pulsatile flow artifacts seen in CSF.

RF Coils

The routine coil of choice for all spinal imaging is the CTL array. This is a receive-only coil typically consisting of six elements in a row with either the upper, middle, or lower four elements separately activated to suit the required imaging section.

Example

Figure 5.8 shows a C-spine image demonstrating trauma.

5.6 ADVANCED APPLICATIONS

Certain advanced brain techniques are now being utilized in the spine. For example, DTI is being used in the spine for pre-surgical planning of tumor resection. Magnetization transfer imaging (see Chapter 1) may be used to show myelin loss.

Chapter 6

Breast

6.1 INTRODUCTION

Breast cancer is the most commonly diagnosed nonskin malignancy in women. Conventional assessment methods such as physical examination and radiographic imaging (ultrasound scan and mammography) have well-known limitations, such as inaccurate differentiation between benign and malignant lesions and estimation of the size of malignant tumors. Furthermore, such conventional assessment is also inaccurate for monitoring neoadjuvant chemotherapy and detection of recurrent tumors. Breast MRI has been shown to have a very high sensitivity for lesion detection and has established a role in equivocal findings from conventional mammography techniques. It is also better at identifying the true extent of cancer when multifocal disease or ductal carcinoma in situ is present. High temporal resolution dynamic contrast-enhanced (DCE) data are often used to improve the specificity of the technique by examining enhancement kinetics. If focal enhancement is present, then post-contrast high-resolution imaging is required to visualize important morphological information. Advanced functional techniques such as MR spectroscopy and diffusion are also beginning to find a place in breast protocols and provide additional information.

Role of MRI

✓ Equivocal mammography/U.S. cases
✓ Radiographically dense breasts
✓ Multifocal disease and ductal carcinoma in situ (DCIS)
✓ Local staging of disease prior to or following neoadjuvant chemotherapy
✓ Screening in certain high risk (e.g., genetic) cases
✓ MR-guided interventions

6.2 CONVENTIONAL TECHNIQUES

Protocols

- *Dynamic contrast-enhanced (DCE) imaging.* This is a fast 2D gradient-echo T_1-weighted sequence with slice coverage traded off to maintain adequate temporal resolution (10–20 s). It is performed bilaterally in the coronal plane or as a single sagittal scan.

Example sequence: FSPGR with TE/TR/flip = 4.2 (in-phase)/10 ms/30°, 35 phases at 9 (coronal) or 4 (sagittal) slices with 5/1 mm thickness/gap.
Coronal scan using a 34 × 17 cm, half-phase (see below) FOV.

- *Alternative "dynamic" 3D volume.* Full breast coverage can be achieved with a 3D volume repeated as fast as possible usually achieving temporal resolutions of around 30–45 s.

Example sequence: FSPGR as above but with a 3D volume slab with between 32–128 slices.

- *Post-contrast high spatial resolution.* 3D volume is usually acquired with fat suppression for a morphological assessment of the tumor. Spatial resolutions should be between 0.3–0.4 mm^2 (in-plane) and 1.5–2.5 mm (through-plane).

Example sequence: as above with TR extended (20 ms) due to fat suppression.

- *Implants.* The type of implant must be known to decide upon sequence. Implants may be single or double lumen containing saline and/or silicon. The pre-scan center frequency must be set accordingly (i.e., center on silicon/water peak for silicon/saline implants, respectively) See Top Tip below.

> Top Tip! Remember when manually adjusting fat suppression or center frequency, the fat peak is to the right (lower frequency) of water. In silicon implants, the silicon peak appears at 100 Hz (at 1.5 T) to the right of fat.

- *T_2-weighted*. This is seldom used in breast imaging.

❖ What is Half-phase Field-of-view?
A bilateral breast scan in the coronal plane is always imaged using a so-called "half-phase" field of view in the SI direction. This is an example of a rectangular FOV, whereby the imaging field of view is reduced in one direction with a concomitant reduction in the matrix size to reduce scan time and maintain resolution. The FOV may also be reduced by other amounts, for example, three-quarter phase.

DCE Analysis

Dynamic images may be viewed in a cine loop or as a single image subtraction of a pre- and a post-contrast time point in order to visualize the area of enhancement. If analysis software is available some simple processing may be performed, for example, pixel-by-pixel parameter maps of percentage enhancement or wash-in rate, graphical analysis, and so on (see Figure 6.2).

RF Coils

Usually a phased-array design, although some surface coils are still in use, operates as receive-only with body coil transmission. Traditionally, the coils have consisted of two closed wells for either single or bilateral breast examinations. More recently open-well designs have been introduced to permit lateral access to either breast for small interventional procedures (see below). The transition to 3.0 Tesla has been slower compared to other coils but these have now become available.

Examples

Figure 6.1 shows an example of a pre- and post-contrast image of a breast tumor, which was found to be a grade 3 invasive carcinoma of no specific type. The tumor can clearly be seen to take up contrast (arrow).

❖ What is Edge Enhancement?
Artifactual enhancement commonly occurs at the edges of the breast in post-processed DCE images (Figure 6.2). This is due to patient motion that has caused the high–low signal interface to move across the image pixel mimicking signal enhancement. Similarly motion-induced

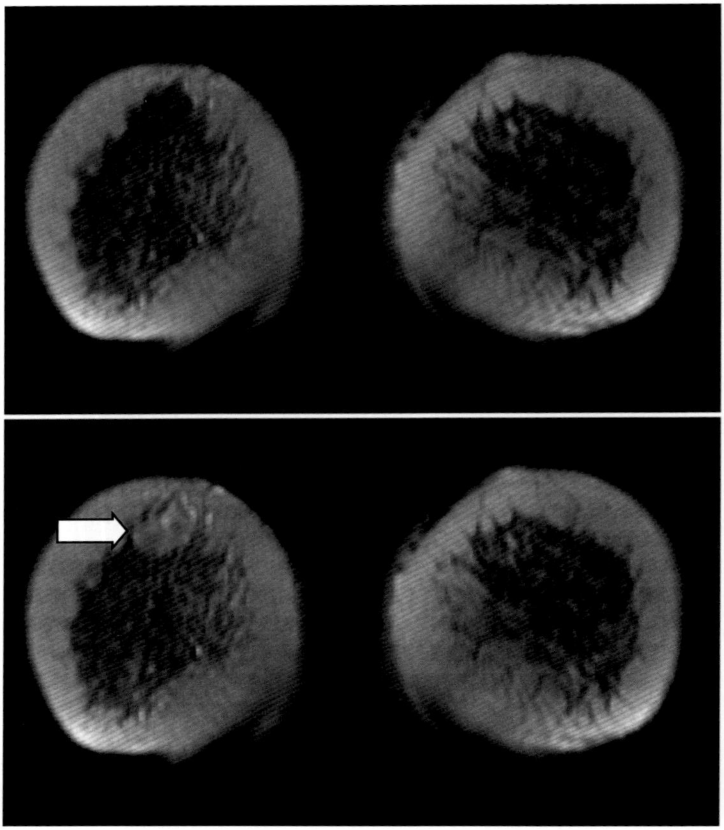

FIGURE 6.1. (top) Pre-contrast breast image in the coronal plane using a FSPGR sequence. (bottom) A post-contrast image at the same slice location. This image illustrates the contrast uptake in the lesion, approximately 20 s after administration of the contrast agent (arrow).

false activation is often seen in functional studies of the brain.

6.3 ADVANCED APPLICATIONS

MR Spectroscopy

Nearly all MRS investigations in the breast have focused on single-voxel techniques. Initial studies examined the diagnostic

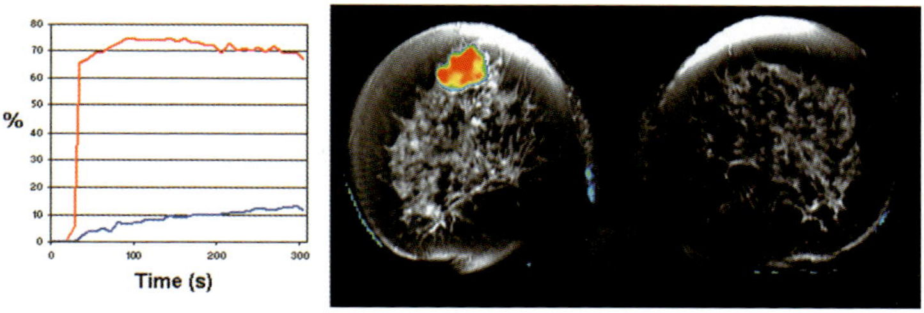

FIGURE 6.2. (left) A plot of signal intensity versus time for two regions of interest: the blue line is taken from a region in normal tissue; the red line corresponds to the tumor. (right) When this is done on a pixel-by-pixel basis an enhancement map can be produced. In this case high enhancement values are displayed in color and overlaid onto greyscale anatomical images.

use of water-to-fat peak ratios. A much more difficult but nevertheless promising method relies on the ability to demonstrate the presence of choline (3.2 ppm), not visible in the normal breast, as a marker for malignancy. Good fat suppression remains the chief hurdle, with the lipid peak readily obscuring the choline resonance. High field MRS may improve matters with increased chemical shift dispersion (peak separation).

Perhaps a more promising role for breast MRS is in the follow-up of chemotherapy. Clinical response based on palpation or imaging depends on tumor size and may take several weeks to demonstrate changes compared to MRS, which may indicate failed response much earlier, thereby optimizing treatment.

Pharmacokinetic Modeling

Much research has focused on fitting the data obtained from DCE to a suitable model to try and obtain physiological information, which may improve the specificity of the technique. In a common *two-compartment* approach, the contrast diffuses from the vascular space into the extracellular–extravascular space according to a rate constant which is a product of the capillary permeability and surface area. The concentration of the agent must be determined at each time point and this necessitates measuring the T_1 relaxation time. To do this on a practical timescale, a heavily proton density-weighted (low flip angle) fast gradient-echo sequence is acquired prior to contrast injection. T_1 is then estimated by comparing the signal obtained in subsequent

T_1-weighted images during the time course of contrast uptake. The application is computationally intensive and the advantage of these models over simpler methods of quantitation remains unproven.

Example sequence: Precede a 2D DCE sequence described above with a single acquisition of FSPGR with TE/TR/flip = 4.2 (in-phase)/10 ms/8°.

Morphological Analysis

Figure 6.3 demonstrates the shapes of a typical benign and malignant lesion highlighted in white on two high-resolution post-contrast images. The benign lesion is smaller and more ovoid compared to the malignant lesion, which has an irregular and spiculated border. Research is being focused on how shape may be quantified to further improve the discrimination of breast tumors and includes parameters such as complexity, circularity, and convexity. Textural analysis based on the variation and distribution of pixel intensities contained within the lesion boundary is also being investigated.

Other Techniques

- *Diffusion-weighted imaging.* This has also been used successfully in the breast to obtain ADC maps of tumors. (For more information see Chapter 5 and Chapter 7, Section 7.7.)

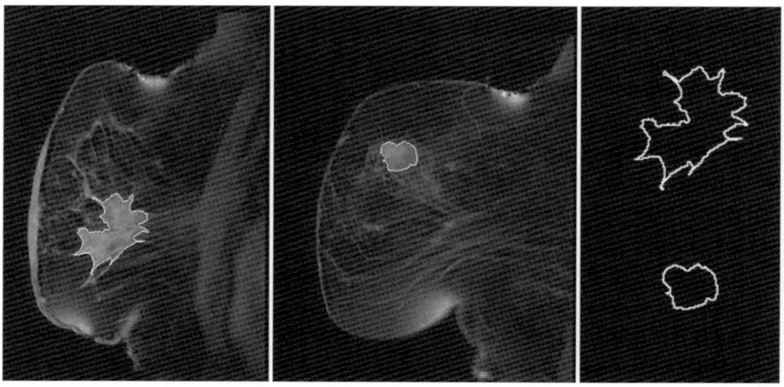

FIGURE 6.3. Examples of the use of post-contrast high-resolution imaging to demonstrate lesion morphology. These contrast-enhanced malignant (left) and benign (middle) lesions have been segmented and their respective shapes are quite different (right).

- *Elastography.* This is a novel technique that attempts to distinguish benign and malignant tumors on the basis of their characteristic tissue stiffness. This development is motivated by the fact that palpation is used to detect breast cancer. It is performed with a device capable of transmitting acoustic shear waves through the tissue and using an imaging sequence, which is sensitive to the propagation of these waves. Typically, a *phase-contrast* type sequence is used which incorporates oscillating motion-sensitive gradients applied in synchronicity with the mechanical device. Elastograms, or parameter maps based on shear stiffness are then calculated and promising results have been produced with good spatial resolution.
- *MR-guided biopsy.* With the adaptation of breast coils to permit open access to either breast the benefits of MR imaging are being increasingly exploited in minor surgical interventions such as needle biopsy and hook-wire localization for lesions that are occult by other diagnostic procedures. The technique is not without its difficulties: moderate to severe susceptibility artifacts (see Chapter 3) are present even with MR-compatible equipment, which depends on field strength and the angulation of the needle with respect to the main field. However, initial work has demonstrated excellent accuracy for lesions larger than 1 cm in diameter.

Chapter 7
Abdomen and Pelvis

7.1 LIVER—INTRODUCTION

The liver, of all of the organs in the abdomen, is the most frequent site of pathology. The detection of extrahepatic disease is as important as detection within the liver itself and MRI is required to provide diagnostic imaging of all the abdominal organs. The introduction of rapid imaging techniques to reduce respiratory artifacts has propelled liver MRI into routine clinical practice and MRI is now the principal modality for the accurate diagnosis of both focal and diffuse liver disease. Furthermore, the advent of new liver-specific contrast agents ensures continued development in this area.

Role of MRI

- ✓ Primary or metastatic tumors
- ✓ Diffuse liver disease (e.g., cirrhosis)
- ✓ Patients with decreased renal function or iodine contrast allergy
- ✓ High-resolution imaging of the gall bladder and biliary tree

7.2 CONVENTIONAL TECHNIQUES

Respiratory Motion

Respiratory motion is an important problem in MRI of the thorax and upper abdomen and various methods exist for its remedy. Respiratory gating monitors the motion of the chest wall with pressure bellows and uses this signal to synchronize the image acquisition with a point in the respiratory cycle with minimum motion. The *TR* is effectively set by the respiration rate, and due to its length, is only suitable for T_2-weighted imaging.

Phase-reordering methods such as ROPE or PEAR, used in T_1-weighted imaging, acquire neighboring lines of *k*-space data at similar stages of the cycle, thereby reducing the artifacts caused by motion. The use of multiple signal averaging (usually four to six) is also a good way of reducing motion artifacts although it extends scan time considerably. Other techniques include navigator echoes (discussed in Chapter 8), or reducing scan times down to a breath-hold (see Ultra-fast Imaging in the Abdomen).

Liver-specific Contrast Agents

Liver-specific contrast agents increase the conspicuity of liver lesions by changing the background signal intensity of the normal liver. They are subdivided into two types: reticulo-endothelial system (RES) agents or hepatocyte-selective agents. The former type are superparamagnetic iron oxides (SPIO; also called ferrumoxides), and these produce a T_2-shortening effect in the reticulo-endothelial cells of the normal liver due to the susceptibility effects of the iron. Lesions therefore appear brighter than normal tissue, which has decreased signal intensity. They typically require long infusion times (30 minutes) but also have a long imaging window compared to extracellular agents.

Manganese-DPDP is the most common hepatocyte agent. These types are T_1-enhancing; that is, normal liver hepatocytes take up the agent and demonstrate an increase in signal intensity so that lesions appear hypointense. Hepatocyte-selective agents are eliminated through the biliary system and also permit the investigation of the biliary tree. (A list of liver agents can be found in Appendix A2.1.)

Protocols

- *Anti-peristaltic agent.* Administration of an antiperistaltic agent (e.g., Buscopan or glucagon) is advised to reduce intestinal motion artifacts.
- *T_1-weighted sequences.* This is the standard fast gradient-echo technique.
- *T_2-weighted sequences.* This is used for lesion detection, breath-hold or respiratory gated.

Example sequence: ssFSE TE/TR = 100/1084 ms with ASSET, 0.58 NEX (partial Fourier) 16 s breath-hold. Slice thickness/gap = 8/2 mm.

Example sequence: FRFSE TE/TR = 121/4286 ms respiratory triggered with ASSET, 3 min 32 s. 6 NEX, Slice thickness/gap = 5/0.5 mm.

- *DCE.* Used for lesion characterization, this is a routine sequence with good temporal resolution. Normal extracelluaIr agents are often used (Gd-DTPA) but new targeted agents are also being exploited.
- *Fat-suppression.* This improves contrast and also removes chemical shift artifacts, which is important in diseases that involve subcapsular parenchyma. It also improves respiratory ghosting, which is mainly due to fat.
- *Out-of-phase gradient-echo.* This is a sequence with fat/water out-of-phase (e.g., OOPS) to detect fatty infiltration of the liver, which is otherwise not discriminated on normal images.

Example

Figure 7.1 shows an axial image of the liver in a normal subject at 3.0 Tesla using a fast-recovery FSE sequence done in a single breath-hold of 21 s.

7.3 ADVANCED APPLICATIONS

Probing Liver Function

- *Hepatic iron concentration.* Relaxation time mapping has been utilized in many applications and is beginning to find a clini-

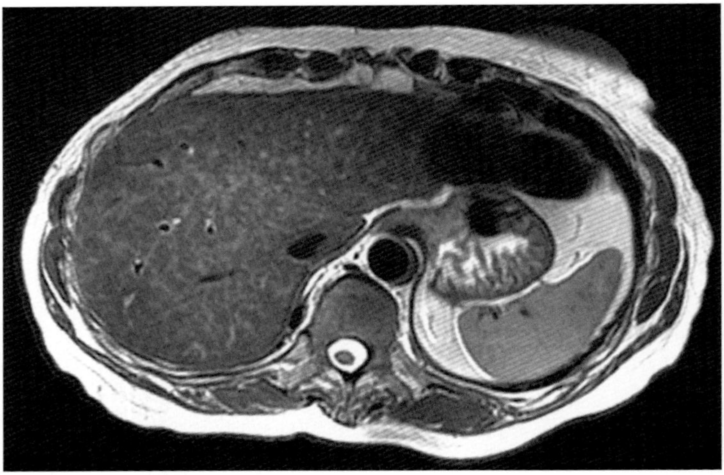

FIGURE 7.1. Fast-recovery FSE scan of the liver in a healthy volunteer at 3.0 Tesla.

cal niche in certain specific areas. In the liver it may be used in cases of "iron-overload", a condition where there is an excessive deposition of iron in the liver, pancreas, and other organs. It has been shown that the transverse relaxation rate R_2 (= $1/T_2$) correlates with hepatic iron content. Multiple images at different echo times are acquired and the signal decay may be fitted to produce pixel-by-pixel maps of R_2. Parallel imaging is used to enable the scans to be performed within a single breath-hold thereby minimizing motion, which produces exaggerated artifacts on the processed images. Some scanners now reconstruct the relaxation time maps as part of a built-in protocol, (usually T_2), but further processing may be needed offline.

- *Multinuclear spectroscopy.* MRS is beginning to be applied to the liver, with both ^{1}H and ^{31}P (phosphorous) single-voxel spectroscopy being used in the evaluation of chronic liver disease. In particular phosphorous spectroscopy has the ability to measure both metabolic information and intracellular pH levels (see below) and has demonstrated changes associated with alcoholic liver disease. Other uses of proton MRS include the quantification of liver fat content in diabetic subjects.

❖ What is Multinuclear Spectroscopy?
MNS or multinuclear spectroscopy refers to investigations of the less commonly studied nuclear spins. Dual-tuned coils are needed, with the resonant frequency set to proton to obtain images for localization and then a different frequency depending on the nucleus of interest. Phosphorous MRS demonstrates excellent dispersion (spread of peaks) and is used to study metabolism. The change in the frequency of the inorganic phosphorous peak can also be used to measure pH.

7.4 MR CHOLANGIOPANCREATOGRAPHY (MRCP)—INTRODUCTION

MRCP is a relatively new application in MRI permitting the noninvasive evaluation of the billiary tract, pancreatic duct, and gall bladder without the risks associated with the gold-standard ERCP (endoscopic retrograde cholangiopancreatography). The basis of the MR protocol is the use of heavily T_2-weighted sequences, which are able to demonstrate the fluid within the lumen, while suppressing signal from surrounding tissues. Both single-slice and multislice techniques work well and recently volume isotropic 3D MRCP has been shown to offer benefits over standard MRCP. In most instances MRCP is now replacing ERCP as a diagnostic tool and a complete examination can be performed in a matter of minutes.

Role of MRI

✓ Screening in patients with low/intermediate choledochlithiasis
✓ Failed or incomplete ERCP
✓ Anomalous ductal anatomy
✓ Post-operative
✓ Primary sclerosing cholangitis (PSC)
✓ Complications of chronic pancreatitis

7.5 CONVENTIONAL TECHNIQUES

Ultrafast Imaging in the Abdomen

The most obvious remedy to chest motion is to get the patient to hold her breath and this is now possible as scan times have decreased with the development of ultrafast imaging sequences. Single-shot techniques such as ssFSE and EPI may be used although the latter is not particularly suited to the abdomen, being prone to susceptibility artifacts from the lungs. Driven equilibrium sequences force longitudinal relaxation, and give good T_2 contrast in shorter times (see Chapter 1). Partial Fourier techniques are also available (HASTE is discussed below). Sometimes two breath-holds are required depending on the coverage, in which case slice ordering is optimized to reduce mispositioning. Perhaps the most important advance in recent times in terms of reducing scan times has been parallel imaging (see Chapter 1).

> Top Tip! Try and intersperse breath-hold scans with non-breath-hold for patients who have difficulty. If this is a real struggle, advise gentle breathing and use multiple signal averages.

Protocols

- *Oral contrast.* Some sites may administer negative contrast agents (e.g., Gastromark) prior to imaging to reduce signal from the bowel.

- *Antiperistaltic agent.* Administration of an antiperistaltic agent (e.g., Buscopan or glucagon) is advised to reduce intestinal motion artifacts.
- *Routine MRCP.* Heavily T_2-weighted imaging (long *TR*) is utilized to show up fluid within ducts. Acquire axial scans covering pancreas and biliary tree with fat suppression. Intermediate echo times can be used to show periductal structures.
- *HASTE or similar.* This is the use of half-scan technique permitting subsecond images to be acquired without motion artifacts or multiple slices within a breath-hold.

Example sequence: single-shot FSE TE/TR = 100/1159 ms 8/2 mm slice thickness, typically 18 images in 20 s, 0.58 NEX (partial Fourier) plus ASSET.

- *Coronal single slice.* This includes three to six radial views of a single slice around the pancreas with 4–7 cm thickness. Using a *TE* = 1000 ms only fluid signal is present producing cholangiogramlike images.

Example sequence: single-shot FSE TE/TR = 1000/2830 ms, 3 views 7 s.

- *3D volume isotropic MRCP.* Good SNR 3D volume with respiratory triggering, this permits reconstruction using MIP (also see Chapter 9).

Example sequence: 3D FSE TE/TR = 145/2857 ms, 28 section slab with 1–2 mm contiguous slices and similar in-plane resolution.

- *Optional T_1-weighted abdomen.* This is used for conventional assessment of surrounding solid organs. Use fast gradient technique with breath-hold, optionally with contrast to demonstrate the viability of the pancreas.

❖ What is HASTE?
HASTE or half-fourier single-shot turbo spin-echo is a partial *k*-space technique. Just over half of the required *k*-space data is collected with the remaining lines reconstructed. This makes it a very rapid sequence, which allows T_2-weighted scans to be acquired in very

short acquisition times reducing susceptibility and motion artifacts. (This sequence is sometimes referred to as "fractional NEX" although it is not related to signal averaging.)

RF Coils

A suitable phased-array body coil should be used to provide optimum signal-to-noise. Development of separate phased-array coils for general abdomen and pelvic imaging continues to be pursued, particularly to meet the challenges of higher field strengths.

Example

Figure 7.2 shows a MIP display from a single-shot TSE sequence using SPIR fat suppression (TE/TR = 260/11716 ms). A stone can clearly be seen in the common bile duct (arrow).

> Top Tip! Reduced signal in a T_2-weighted MRCP scan may be down to a normal lack of fluid in the ducts rather than a poor imaging sequence.

7.6 ADVANCED APPLICATIONS

Real-time

Ultrafast snapshot techniques are finding increasing application as a method of producing real-time imaging (see also Chapter 8). MRCP is an example of an area which may benefit from this advancement, where a potential use is the rapid localization of planes of interest.

7.7 PROSTATE—INTRODUCTION

The prostate gland is an inverted pyramid that lies inferior to the neck of the bladder. It consists of three regions, an outer peripheral zone, which appears hyperintense on T_2-weighted images and inner central and transition zones, which are not readily distinguished on MRI and usually referred to as a combined central gland.

Prostate cancer is now the most commonly occurring malignancy in men. Currently no single test or imaging modality can accurately diagnose and stage prostate cancer. MRI has demonstrated higher accuracy than other imaging modalities in assess-

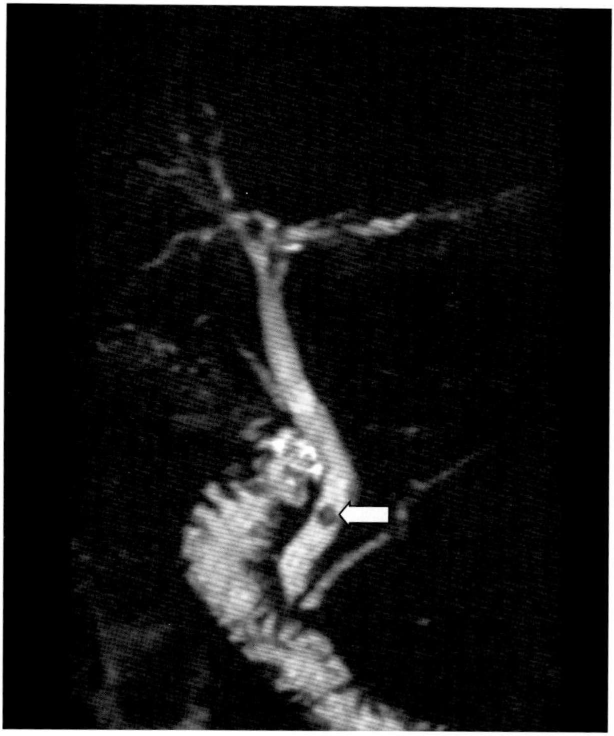

FIGURE 7.2. This MRCP examination displayed as a MIP shows a stone in the common bile duct.

ing seminal vesicle invasion and extracapsular extension. Sensitivity within the gland is also high although the low specificity of tumor hypointensity within the peripheral zone is further reduced for the relatively smaller number of lesions which occur in the central gland. This has led to the utilization of less routine MRI techniques, specifically, dynamic contrast enhancement (DCE) and MR spectroscopy, both of which have been shown to provide complementary information.

Role of MRI

✓ Mainly used in staging and localization of disease
✓ Post-radiotherapy/surgical recurrence

✓ Diagnosis only in a few highly selected patients
✓ Pre-treatment radiotherapy planning

7.8 CONVENTIONAL TECHNIQUES

Protocols

- *Antiperistaltic agent.* Administration of an antiperistaltic agent (e.g., Buscopan or glucagon) is advised to reduce intestinal motion artifacts.
- *Post-treatment.* A three-week period should be observed following radiotherapy or surgery to minimize effect on MR appearance.
- *Sagittal plane.* This is used as a localizer but is also helpful to identify inner/outer gland and anterior fibromuscular stroma.
- *Axial T_2–W.* This includes whole pelvis coverage, from bifurcation of the aorta downwards. It is necessary for accurate staging, that is, visualization of pelvic wall and pelvic lymph nodes.

Example sequence: FSE TE/TR = 100–140/4500 ms, FOV = 24–30 cm, 5/1 mm slices.

- *Axial T_2–W (small FOV).* This covers seminal vesicles and the prostate gland and gives an excellent depiction of internal zonal anatomy and gold standard for staging.

Example sequence: as above with FOV reduced to 14–18 cm and 3/0 mm slices.

- *T_2–W coronal.* As above, this defines lateral margins and demonstrates the apex and base of gland/seminal vesicles. These images are excellent at 3.0 Tesla.
- *T_1-weighted.* Dynamic contrast-enhancement may be used routinely in some medical centers. Reasonable temporal and spatial resolution is required.

Example sequence: FSPGR with TE/TR/flip = 4.2 (in-phase)/10 ms/30°, 35 phases at 4 (axial) slices with 7/2 mm.

RF Coils

For optimum SNR an endorectal (ER) surface coil may be used either alone or in conjunction with a surface coil placed on the abdomen to improve signal anterior to the gland. ER coils are usually inflatable balloon-types, which also act to fix the prostate and reduce motion, but rigid probes have also been used. Images suffer from signal flair, which may be resolved with intensity correction (see below). Alternatively, and to avoid patient discomfort, a pelvic phased-array coil may be used comprising posterior and anterior elements, the latter of which may be strapped to the abdomen to reduce motion. For spectroscopy, the ER coil must be used to boost the inherently low SNR. At high field excellent image quality can be obtained by using a flexible array coil only.

Examples

Figure 7.3 shows two axial T_2-weighted images acquired using an ER coil. The image on the left shows the normal high signal intensity fluid of the seminal vesicles. The image on the right is taken through the prostate gland and shows enlargement of the gland due to benign prostatic hyperplasia (BPH). The neurovascular bundles that lie posterolateral to the gland are best visualized with an ER coil. However, in both these images there is considerable signal flair due to the proximity of the prostate to the ER coil.

Excellent image quality can be obtained at higher field strengths without using an ER coil (Figure 7.4). A focus of low signal intensity indicative of cancer can be seen in both these images acquired at 3.0 Tesla.

❖ What is Intensity Correction?
Intensity correction algorithms (e.g., SCIC) may be used to improve the B_1 inhomogeneity caused by the use of surface coils. This signal variation is particularly evident in the prostate when an ER coil is used. Post-processing improves this by normalizing the coil sensitivity profile, often utilizing a low-contrast proton density-weighted image, which readily demonstrates the B_1 inhomogeneity of the coil.

7.9 ADVANCED APPLICATIONS

MR Spectroscopy

Spectroscopy has been used in the prostate successfully for a number of years as a research tool. Initially work focused on single-voxel MRS in order to measure citrate (2.6 ppm) as a marker for carcinoma and improve the specificity of T_2-weighted hyperintensity. In the last few years much interest has been shown in developing MRSI in the prostate-to map the distribu-

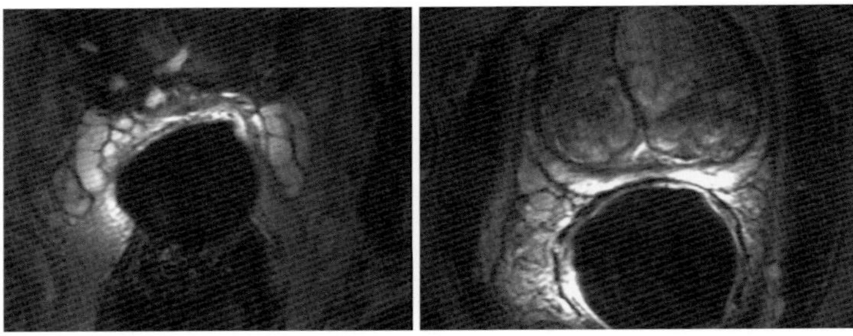

FIGURE 7.3. Axial T_2-weighted images of seminal vesicles (left), and prostate gland (right) in a patient with BPH and acquired with an endorectal coil at 1.5 Tesla.

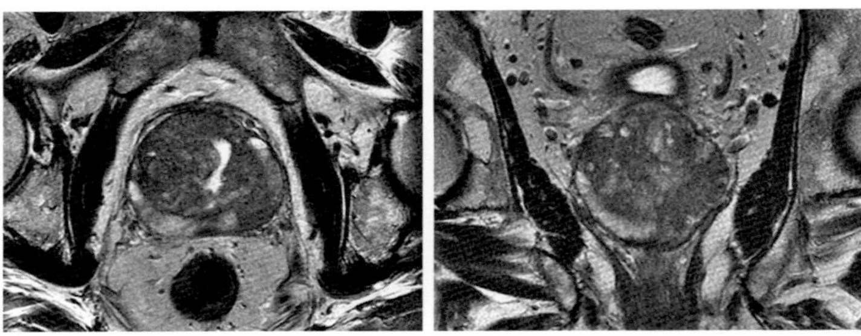

FIGURE 7.4. Axial (left) and coronal (right) T_2-weighted images at 3.0 Tesla using a torso coil.

tions of citrate-to-choline (and/or creatine) ratios across the gland.

Sequences have been developed specifically for the prostate (e.g., PROSE), which use *spectral–spatial* pulses to reduce lipid contamination. The technique has been successfully used to demonstrate recurrence in post-surgical and radiotherapy cases.

Diffusion

Tumor growth causes an increase in cellularity resulting in a restriction of the diffusion of water molecules. This can be readily measured using diffusion-weighted sequences in much the same way as in the brain (see Chapter 5). Although the technique is more challenging in the prostate, with SNR being much

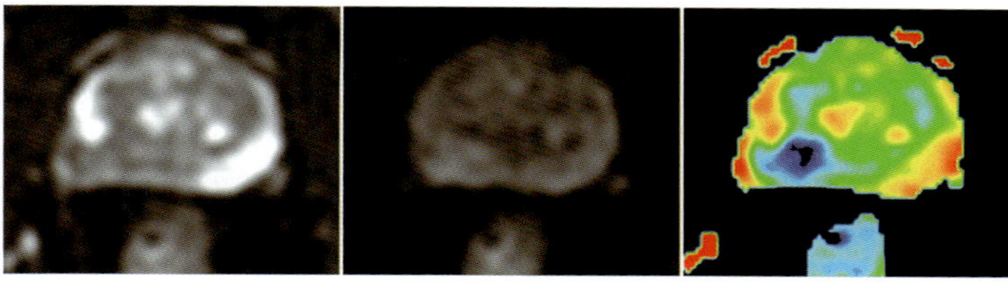

FIGURE 7.5. Example of the use of DWI in prostate cancer. Images are (left to right) DWI with $b = 0$, $b = 700\,\mathrm{s/mm^2}$, and ADC map.

poorer, good results have been obtained and reduced ADC values have been demonstrated in tumors.

Figure 7.5 shows example images from a DWI study of the prostate. The first two images are EPI scans acquired with diffusion gradients of $b = 0$ and $b = 700\,\mathrm{s/mm^2}$ and the third image on the right shows a color map of ADC calculated from the previous two images. A region in the right peripheral zone demonstrates lower (blue) values of ADC compared to the normally high values (red/orange). Diffusion tensor studies are also being investigated in the prostate although this work is still in its infancy.

Radiotherapy Planning

Advanced radiotherapy delivery techniques such as IMRT (intensity modulated radiotherapy) are able to produce highly conformal treatments thereby improving tumor control and reducing complications. This requires images with improved soft-tissue contrast such as MRI to be incorporated into the planning. MRI is finding a role in the radiotherapy planning of the prostate utilizing both routine and advanced techniques for improving the visualization of tumor and normal anatomy. Because registration with CT data is paramount, issues such as patient positioning and geometric distortion need to be addressed. Usually, a flat board is placed on the scanner bed to replicate treatment set-up and distortion minimized using high-bandwidth scans or corrected with post-processing.

7.10 GYNECOLOGY—INTRODUCTION

Over the last few years MRI has established itself as an important imaging modality for the evaluation of the female pelvis. Uterine zonal anatomy and temporal changes are well demonstrated on T_2-weighted images. Staging of endometrial and cervical carcinoma with MRI is superior to other imaging modalities. In the evaluation of ovarian tumors, experience is less established. However, the introduction of 3.0 Tesla scanners into clinical practice and the improvements in image quality allow an increasingly accurate evaluation of pelvic pathologies and continue to drive its utilization in this area.

Role of MRI

✓ Evaluation of benign pathology
  ○ Uterus (endometrial, polyps/hyperplasia, endometriosis, adenomyosis, fibroids)
  ○ Fallopian tubes and ovary (cysts, salphingo-oophoritis, cystadenomas)

✓ Evaluation of primary gynecological malignancy (and staging)
  ○ Vulval and vaginal tumor
  ○ Cervical tumor
  ○ Uterus (myometrial, endometrial tumors)
  ○ Ovarian tumor

✓ Monitoring tumor response to chemotherapy

✓ Evaluation of recurrent malignant disease

7.11 CONVENTIONAL TECHNIQUES

Protocols

- *Antiperistaltic agent.* Administration of an antiperistaltic agent (e.g., Buscopan or glucagon) is advised to reduce intestinal motion artifacts.
- *Sagittal and axial T_2–W.*

Example sequence: FSE TE/TR = 120/3280 ms 3/1 mm 24 cm FOV with 256 × 224 matrix.

- *Coronal oblique T_2–W.* Commonly perpendicular to the uterine cavity and/or cervical cavity, this sequence gives axial views with respect to the uterus or cervix.
- *Additional sequences.* These are obtained depending upon the indication.
  - ○ T_1–*W* sequence is obtained, for example, to demonstrate hemorrhagic ovarian cystic fluid.

Example sequence: FSE TE/TR = 10/480 ms 5/2 mm 24 cm FOV with 256 × 224 matrix.

 - T_1–*W* fat-saturated sequence allows the diagnosis of dermoid tumours of ovaries.
 - Axial ssFSE through the abdomen is routinely acquired in all cases of neoplastic lesions to demonstrate/rule out other pathology.
- *Contrast*. Dynamic imaging is rarely used. However, a 3D FSPGR volume post-contrast is sometimes acquired in vaginal/vulva tumors showing excellent detail from surrounding structures.
- *Saturation bands*. These may be placed both anteriorly and posteriorly to reduce signal flare from body wall fat, and respiratory ghosting.

RF Coils

A flexible multichannel phased-array coil should be used in combination with the body coil, with the coil strapped to the pelvis. In certain instances, for example, extremely obese patients or those with abdominal protuberances, the body coil has to be used on its own due to limited signal depth of surface coils. There has been little evidence to suggest any advantages of using endocavity coils and certainly at high field, these are unnecessary as image quality is excellent.

Examples

Figure 7.6 illustrates a common problem encountered in pelvic and abdominal imaging at 3.0 Tesla. The images are from patients with an ovarian cyst (top left), and a carcinoma of the ovary (top right) using a T_2-weighted FSE-XL sequence. In both these images there is a marked drop of signal towards the anterior caused by the increased dielectric effect at high field. This is remedied in the corresponding images shown below by using a so-called dielectric pad, placed on top of the abdomen, which reduces the effect and improves signal homogeneity.

> Top Tip! Use a dielectric pad placed on the abdomen to reduce signal inhomogeneity in pelvis/abdomen imaging at high field.

❖ What is a Dielectric Pad?
At high RF frequencies (beyond 100 MHz) the behavior of the B_1 field within the patient causes inhomogeneity of

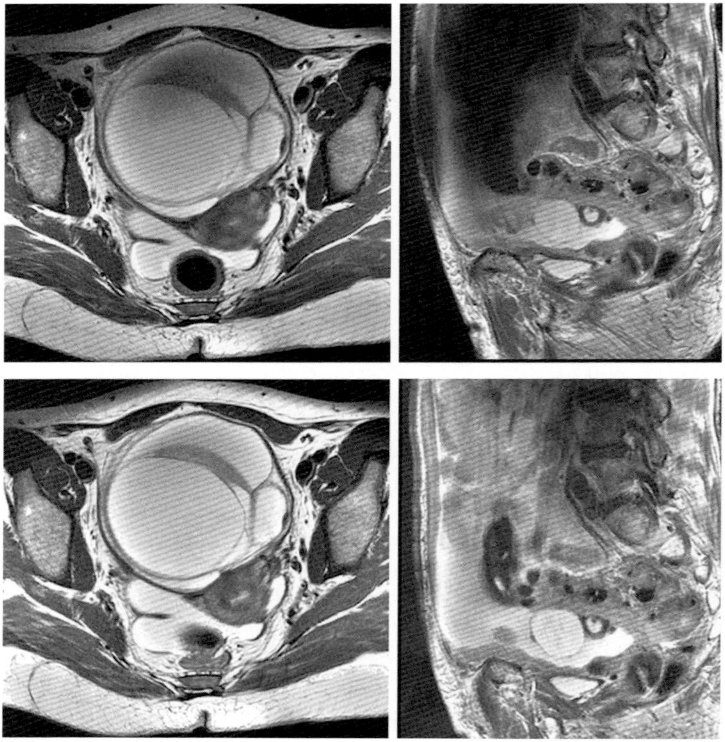

FIGURE 7.6. 3.0 Tesla images of the ovary (top) illustrate the problem associated with the increased dielectric effect at high field. There is considerable signal drop anteriorly, which is rectified in the corresponding images (below) by using a dielectric pad.

signal intensity due to a variety of conductive and dielectric effects. This results in increase and decrease of signal at the center and periphery of an object, respectively. The B_1 distortion may be manipulated by using appropriately placed material (dielectric pads) with high dielectric constants, pulling the high signal areas towards the material and improving overall homogeneity. A bag of water, doped appropriately (e.g., $MnCl_2$) so it does not appear in the image, works well.

7.12 ADVANCED APPLICATIONS

MR Spectroscopy

Initial work has involved using 2D MRSI in ovarian tumors with spectra demonstrating choline, creatine, and N-acetyl metabolites.

Chapter 8
Cardiac MRI

8.1 INTRODUCTION

Cardiovascular disease is now the leading cause of death in industrialized countries. Early cardiac MRI was limited due to lack of fast scanning and difficulties associated with cardiac and respiratory motion. Today, dedicated solutions at both a hardware and software level have transformed cardiac MRI into a state-of-the-art imaging modality of choice. It is able to provide not only morphological imaging but also functional assessment of the cardiac pump and is used to evaluate myocardial perfusion and viability. Cardiac MRI is now the best method of estimating ventricular volume and has developed a role for investigating anomalous coronary arteries and coronary plaques.

Role of MRI

- ✓ Angiography (including pulmonary)
- ✓ Valvular heart disease
- ✓ Myocardial infarction/viability/stress testing
- ✓ Congenital heart disease
- ✓ Anomalous coronary arteries—between aortic root and pulmonary artery/right ventricular outflow tract
- ✓ Coarction, aneurysm
- ✓ Arrhythmogenic right ventricular dysplasia, hypertrophic and dilated cardiomyopathy (ECG diagnosed)
- ✓ Cardiac masses, obesity
- ✓ Sarcoidosis
- ✓ Thalassemia

8.2 CONVENTIONAL TECHNIQUES

ECG Gating

Gating is required for all cardiac scans to reduce motion artifacts by synchronizing the pulse sequence with the periodicity of the heart. Gating ensures that each phase-encoding step is acquired at the same phase of the cardiac cycle. It is achieved by monitoring the R–R interval from the ECG output, or sometimes from a peripheral pulse (via a photosensitive transducer on the fingernail). The patient's heartrate determines the effective *TR*, adjusted slightly by a delay period to account for any fluctuations. The R-wave is chosen as the gating signal because it has the highest peak and is easily detectable. An image obtained just after the R-wave is an end-diastole image, at a time when the ventricular chambers are most dilated.

Retrospective gating acquires images continually and records the ECG trace to enable *k*-space to be filled in afterwards with selected data.

> Top Tip! If the ECG trace is poor it is worth spending a few minutes repositioning the ECG leads rather than continuing.

Myocardial Tagging

This technique is used to monitor cardiac wall thickness and motion. Magnetization is deliberately saturated in a regular pattern across the image so that it appears darker than the surrounding tissue. This provides fiducial markers or *tag-lines* within the tissue itself and can be imposed as either parallel lines or a square grid, which move with the tissue and permit the visualization of motion defects and myocardial strain. In conventional techniques (SPAMM), the darkness of the tags gradually reduces due to T_1 recovery during the cardiac cycle and this is improved in modified implementations such as CSPAMM.

Cine MRI

Cine MRI refers to any fast multiphase technique that can be used to acquire images which when played back represent the heart in motion. It has been shown to be useful in quantifying ventricular morphology and function. Scan times may be kept short enough to permit breath-hold imaging (<20 s), whereby the chest motion and heart position are fixed throughout the acquisition, permitting multiphase imaging at the several locations.

Short axis views through the left ventricle can be used to draw the end systolic and end diastolic volumes (ESV and EDV) manually, requiring at least 16 phases. The ejection fraction (EF) may then be calculated as the relative increase in volume.

Segmented *k*-space techniques are now used to reduce imaging to a 16-cycle breath-hold, and when combined with ultrafast gradient-echo techniques (EPI, HASTE, and trueFISP) this can be further reduced to 2 to 4 cycles.

Perfusion and Viability Imaging

Myocardial perfusion imaging provides better resolution than with either SPECT or PET without the disadvantage of radiation dose. First-pass contrast-enhanced images are acquired using a fast gradient sequence (usually inversion prepared to improve T_1-weighting) with ischemic regions within the cardiac muscle showing up as signal defects. Imaging the heart under stress demonstrates infarcts more readily, and a practical alternative to imaging under physical stress is to administer some pharmacological form of stress. Commonly dobutamine or adenosine is used which acts as a vasodilator to demonstrate hemodynamically significant stenoses, and differences between the rest and stress images are compared.

Delayed contrast enhancement is used to assess cardiac viability. In this case, late hyperenhancement (rather than first-pass hypoenhancement), due to impaired wash-out, can predict the degree of damage in the dysfunctioning myocardium.

Protocols

- *General.* ECG gating is essential plus some method of respiratory compensation or breath-hold is desirable.
- *Short axis view.* This is good for visualizing wall thickness/motion and myocardial perfusion.
- *Black-blood.* This uses spin-echo sequences for morphological information. There is good blood/tissue contrast but limited temporal resolution. Inversion pulses (see below) can be used to overcome disordered flow.

Example sequence:FSE-XL TE/TR = 44/1644 ms with 256 × 224 matrix, 8 mm slice with a 37 × 26 cm FOV.

- *Cine sequence.* This is a short *TR* gradient-echo sequence producing bright-blood images. It is used to provide dynamic views of the cardiac cycle (see Figure 8.2).

Example sequence: FSPGR TE/TR/flip = 3.4/5.8 ms/12° using 8/2 mm slices and a matrix of 256 × 160–192 with 39 × 31 cm FOV.
A total of 20 phases at 5–6 locations.

- *Tagged imaging.* This includes parallel or grid tag-lines, typically covering eight slices and eight phases (see Figure 8.4).

Example sequence: FGR TE/TR/flip = 2.2/4.6 ms/12°, scan time of 27 s.

- *Inversion recovery.* This is the use of a double inversion pulse to null blood and fat signal creating black-blood images with the blood-myocardial interface more clearly visualized.

Example sequence: FSE as above with inversion recovery.

- *Delayed contrast-enhanced imaging.* Use T_1–W fast gradient-echo with inversion recovery. Optimize TI (160–250 ms) in relation to time following injection for myocardium suppression. It is used to assess myocardial viability 10–15 min post-injection.
- *Coronary MRA.* Localization is the main issue, requiring a good four-chamber view. Good fat suppression and triggering are also essential. It is usually performed on dedicated cardiac scanners.

RF Coils

Most cardiac work is performed well enough with standard body or phased-array coils, although dedicated cardiac coils are also available. All coils should have separate multichannel elements capable of parallel imaging for the required acquisition speed.

Examples

One of the difficulties associated with cardiac MRI is determining the correct imaging plane prescription to obtain short/long axis and four-chamber views of the heart. A schematic diagram demonstrating image plane orientations is given in Figure 8.1.

Figure 8.2 shows two images taken from a FSPGR cine acquisition demonstrating a short axis view of the left ventricle during systole and diastole. A total of 20 phases at five slice locations was acquired using this sequence.

A four-chamber view is acquired from scans aligned parallel to a line connecting the center of the left ventricle cavity and the apex of the right ventricle (see Figure 8.1(d) and (e)). The single slice image in Figure 8.3 shows the interrelationships of the ventricles and atria and a cine view may be used to demonstrate the aortic and mitral valves.

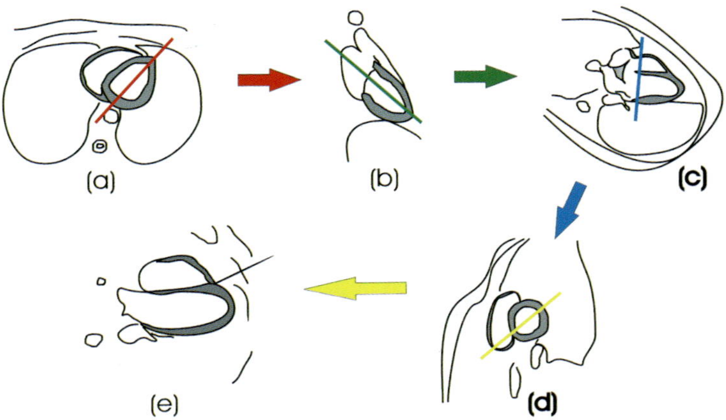

FIGURE 8.1. Diagrammatic representation of image plane prescription in cardiac MRI: (a) axial, (b) two-chamber view, (c) nearly four-chamber, (d) short axis and, (e) four-chamber long axis.

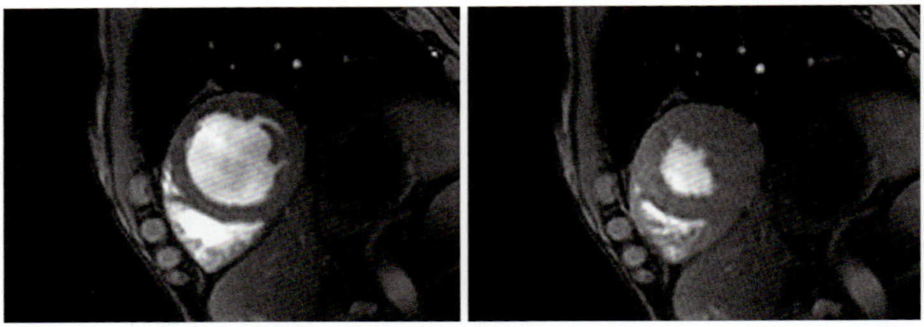

FIGURE 8.2. Short axis views of the left ventricle during diastole (left) and systole (right).

An example of cardiac spin-tagging is shown in Figure 8.4 acquired in a healthy volunteer. Here a grid pattern is used to monitor wall motion. The tag-line deformation illustrates the contraction and rotation of the heart that occurs between these two images taken at different phases of the cardiac cycle. In patients, a lack of pattern distortion indicates nonfunctioning myocardium.

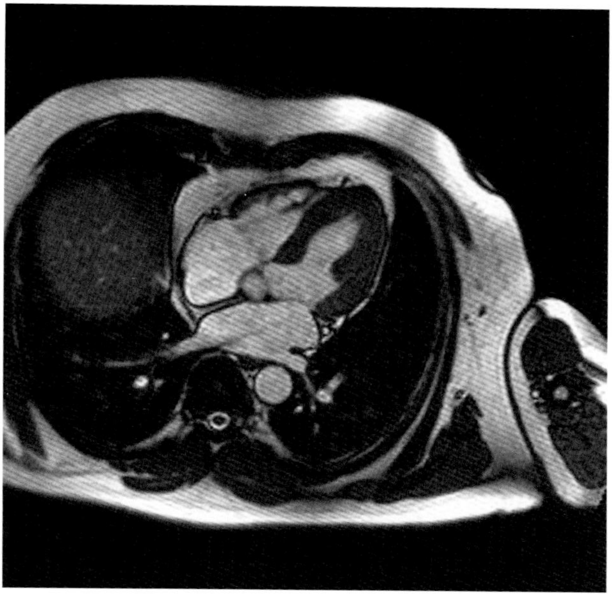

FIGURE 8.3. Four-chamber view of the heart demonstrating the relationships of the ventricles and atria.

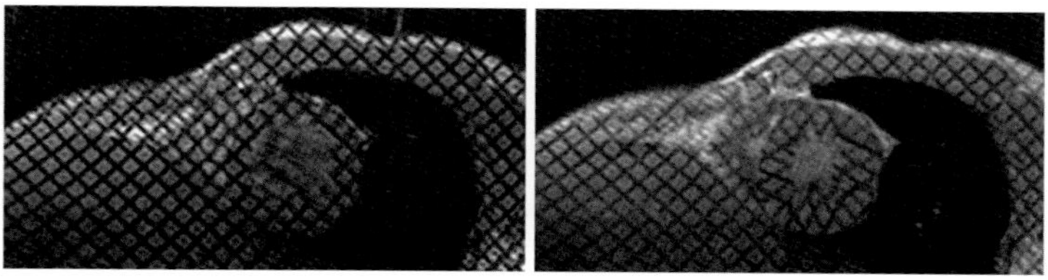

FIGURE 8.4. Spin-tagging using grid tags to visualize cardiac wall motion.

8.3 ADVANCED APPLICATIONS

Real-time: MR-echo

Combining ultrafast gradient sequences with spiral *k*-space trajectories, faster image processing, and temporal interpolation means that real-time cardiac MRI is now feasible. This development is particularly useful in patients unable to hold their breath or with arrhythmias. New techniques (e.g., *k-t* BLAST) are being introduced that can drastically cut acquisition times down, imaging at a rate between 30 and 70 frames per second. This provides the ability to dynamically study all forms of physiological motion and provides cardiac data, which is comparable to echocardiography.

Navigator Echoes

Navigator echoes are used generally to compensate for physiological motion. Although they have been used in research for many years they are only now beginning to find their way onto clinical scanners. They work by using a pre-pulse, which acquires data at an area perpendicular to a moving structure. Usually, the high–low signal interface of the diaphragm is chosen to monitor respiratory movement. This produces a much more accurate method of synchronizing image data to the respiratory conditions of the patient and can be used in conjunction with other methods to restrict imaging over a certain diaphragm displacement "window" or even retrospectively in post-acquisition correction methods. It is more accurate than other gating techniques and requires no sensing equipment. The technique has wide applications but in cardiac work it is used in 3D coronary artery imaging where long scan times prohibit breath-holding. Adaptive approaches utilize navigator detection to perform real-time adjustments of the imaging plane.

MR Spectroscopy

Another potential method for assessing myocardial viability is phosphorous MRS. A decrease in phosphocreatine (PCr) and an increase in inorganic phosphorous (Pi) occurs within seconds of reduced oxygen supply (also see What Is Multinuclear Spectroscopy?, Chapter 7).

Chapter 9
MR Angiography

9.1 INTRODUCTION

MRI is extremely sensitive to motion and flow often leading to undesirable artifacts. These effects are used advantageously in MR angiography (MRA) to visualize the vascular anatomy. Generally techniques are referred to as being either "black-blood" or "white-blood" depending on whether moving spins produce signal, which is darker or brighter than stationary tissue. In addition contrast enhancement is now being used on a routine basis to provide direct imaging of the vascular tree.

MRA provides a noninvasive alternative to conventional catheter angiography and is free from the risks of iodinated contrast and arterial puncture. MRA is widely used for intracranial arteries and in the carotid arteries, which are a common site of atherosclerosis resulting in a reduction of cerebral flow. It is also useful in investigating disease in the aorta, renal and pulmonary arteries, as well as peripheral supply. Additionally it is used to screen patients with a history of aneurysm.

Thanks to higher field strengths, new standards of image detail are being set, with spatial resolutions down to $0.4 \times 0.4 \times 0.6$ mm permitting the demonstration of ever more distal vessels.

Role of MRI

✓ Intracranial
✓ Carotids
✓ Pulmonary and coronary
✓ Abdominal aorta and renal
✓ Peripheral
✓ MR venography

9.2 CONVENTIONAL TECHNIQUES

Time-of-flight (TOF)

Time-of-flight techniques describe phenomena such as high-velocity signal loss and in-flow enhancement, although the term is more commonly reserved for the latter.

High-velocity signal loss leads to the phenomenon of black-blood in a spin-echo sequence. Spins moving between the 90° and 180° pulses are not refocused, as is the case for stationary spins, so their signal is attenuated.

In-flow enhancement is a gradient-echo effect, in which spins moving into the imaged slice appear brighter than tissue within the slice, which have received repeated RF pulses. The moving spins have not experienced these RF pulses and the signal is higher than the saturated (constant) signal from the imaged slice (white-blood). Due to the progressive saturation of the flowing spins, the effect can only be exploited over a limited slice thickness. Sequences like TONE compensate for this by using variable flip angles across the slice profile.

Black-blood techniques have some advantages: they are less prone to susceptibility artifacts, and there is less over-estimation of stenosis caused by turbulent flow.

> Top Tip! Always prescribe TOF slices against the direction of flow: for example, for arterial blood in circle of willis, start at the top and work downwards to reduce through-plane saturation.

Phase-contrast (PC-MRA)

This technique uses a bipolar gradient scheme, which sensitizes the sequence to flow. Gradients of equal amplitude and opposite polarity produce an identical dephasing and rephasing of the stationary spins, whereas moving spins can be discriminated by their change of phase that depends on the velocity of motion. The amplitude of the gradients is adjusted by the *velocity encoding* (VENC) parameter, which sets the maximum velocity that can be distinguished by the sequence, and needs to be appropriately selected. In practice separate images with velocity gradients in each orthogonal direction are used so that an image sensitive to flow direction can be obtained. PC-MRA has the advantage that only flowing spins contribute to the signal (whereas short T_1 tissue will appear as flow in TOF) and is particularly useful for slow-flow. It has been mainly applied in renal MRA but is used less often nowadays.

> Top Tip! Try a series of short 2D PC-MRAs with a variety of VENC values to establish the correct value before acquiring the longer 3D sequence.

Contrast-enhanced MRA

Contrast-enhanced MRA (CE-MRA) combines the use of fast 3D gradient-echo techniques with the intravenous injection of a suitable contrast agent. The T_1-shortening of the contrast agent is used to observe the blood directly. Unlike TOF there is no saturation effect to limit the volume coverage and it works equally well in any plane. CE-MRA is particularly useful in peripheral MRA (see below) where prohibitively long acquisition times and pulsatile flow limit the usefulness of TOF techniques.

Currently, normal extracellular contrast agents are being used. *Gadovist* (Gd-DO3A-butriol, or Gadobutrol) is a new agent suited to CE-MRA as it can be used in higher concentrations for better visualization of small vessels. In addition, some specific blood pool agents are now undergoing clinical trials (see Chapter 1 and Appendix A2.1).

Stepping Table Technique

Peripheral MRA requires coverage from the renal arteries down to the pedal arteries. Usually this is performed as a "bolus chase" technique whereby post-contrast 3D acquisitions are collected at three or more separate locations or *stations* while the patient table is moved, giving it the alternative name of *stepping table* MRA. Often a dedicated RF coil is used for the extremities to provide sufficient spatial resolution. Pre-contrast "mask" images are acquired at each station in order to display subtracted data at the end.

Protocols

- *2D or 3D TOF Head.* This is used for carotids and/or circle of Willis and consists of multiple thin slices or a whole volume fast-gradient sequence. It is processed using MIPs as part of sequence (see below).

Example sequence: FSPGR with TE/TR/flip = 3.4/21 ms/15°, FOV 22 × 16 cm (384 × 224), slice thickness 1 mm.

- *Peripheral MRA.* This is a bolus-chase contrast-enhanced technique. Three stations (top, middle, and bottom) are acquired using a body coil for the first two and a phased-array coil around the legs for the lower station.

Example sequence: Gradient-echo with TE/TR/flip = 1.5–2.0/4–5 ms/20–25°, 384 × 192 matrix increasing to 512 × 288 for middle and lower stations, slice thickness 3.2/–2.4 (overlap) mm for top, 2.8/–2.1 (middle) and 2.4/–1.8 (lower) See Figure 9.4.

- *Renal.* This necessitates use of parallel imaging to get good temporal resolution plus phased-array coil.

Example sequence: FGRE with TE/TR/flip = 1.2/9.4 ms/45°, 320 × 160 matrix and slice thickness 2.6/–1.3 mm.

RF Coils

Routine RF coils may be used as appropriate but dedicated coils are also now available for certain anatomical areas to improve SNR. For example, combined head and neck neurovascular coils may be used, comprising a head coil with a detachable anterior neck element.

For peripheral work, phased arrays can be used for lower abdomen and lower extremity studies with 126 cm superior–inferior coverage. Some vendors now offer a "trouser coil" specifically for this purpose producing a fifteenfold increase in signal compared to a standard body coil. A further approach is to fix a phased array to the scanner bed and move the patient through it by means of a separate board.

Analysis and Display of 3D Data

By far the most common post-processing technique used in MRA is the *Maximum Intensity Projection* algorithm or MIP. This uses a method of raytracing, whereby the maximum pixel intensity along the path of a set of mathematical rays cast through the volume data is displayed in the final image. Analogous to this is the *minimum intensity projection* (denoted mIP) for black-blood techniques. Usually the MIP is shown as a *shaded surface display,* which reduces the volume data to a segmented surface to which lighting is added to enhance visualization. As with any general 3D MRI, the data can also be reconstructed in *multiplanar reformats* (MPR) to view the data in any arbitrary plane.

Top Tip! Always interrogate the original raw data as MIPs can be prone to artifacts, for example, discontinuities at the edges of separate slabs caused by differences in saturation or movement (see also MOTSA and CHARM).

Examples

An example of PC-MRA is shown in Figure 9.1 investigating possible thrombosis in the transverse sinus. In this situation the expected slow-flow makes PC-MRA the preferred technique. CE-MRA cannot be used due to the enhancing nature of blood clots.

Figure 9.2 illustrates a MIP taken from a TOF examination of the circle of Willis. Rapid venous return makes the use of contrast agents problematic in this area and TOF is often used to produce optimum images with excellent spatial resolution.

In carotid examinations the TOF technique is limited in the region of bifurcation as turbulent flow creates intervoxel dephas-

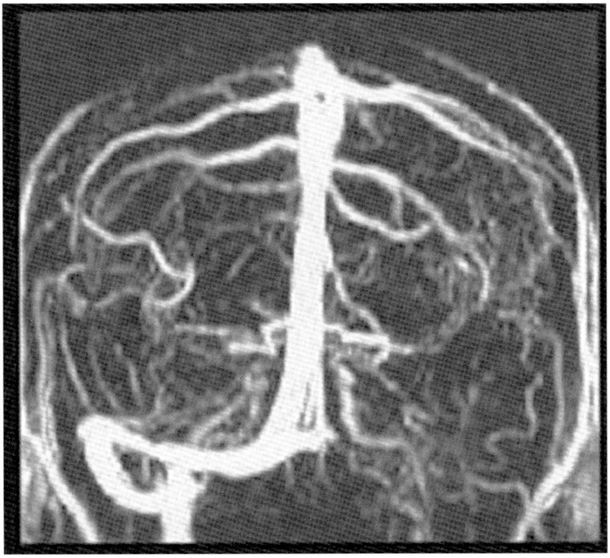

FIGURE 9.1. A phase-contrast venogram of the sagittal and transverse sinus.

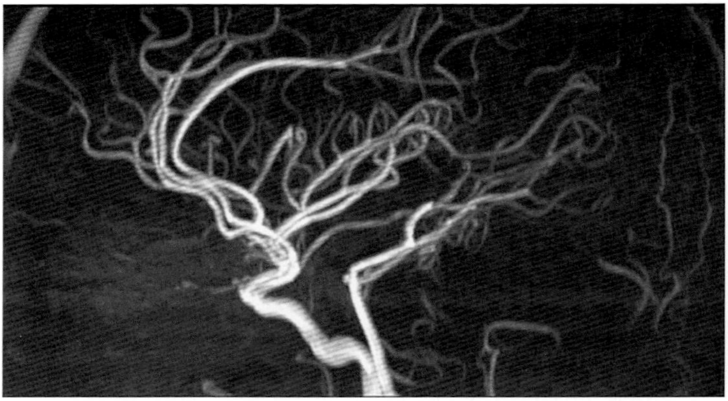

FIGURE 9.2. An example of a 3D TOF angiogram of the circle of Willis, which has been displayed using a maximum intensity projection (MIP).

ing which over-emphasizes any stenosis. For a complete investigation CE-MRA is the preferred choice. An example is demonstrated in Figure 9.3 with coverage of the vascular tree from the aortic arch to the intracranial vessels. This scan was used to investigate an acute cerebral infarct.

Finally, Figure 9.4 (left) demonstrates a peripheral MRA study acquired using three separate stations covering the aorto–illiac arteries, femoral arteries, and the popliteal–tibial arteries, respectively. The three volumes have been processed as MIPs and displayed with an inverted greyscale to provide a comparison with conventional DSA. In this example there is a stenosis in the left external iliac artery (inset shows magnified view of the reduced flow) and the internal iliac also appears affected. There is also increased collateral flow in the vessels further down the left side.

The stepping table technique can also be used in whole-body screening (Figure 9.4, right) where head-to-knee coverage is required.

9.3 ADVANCED APPLICATIONS

Bolus and Sequence Timing in CE-MRA

The crucial aspect in producing good quality CE-MRA is timing the contrast bolus so it arrives in the vessels of interest as the

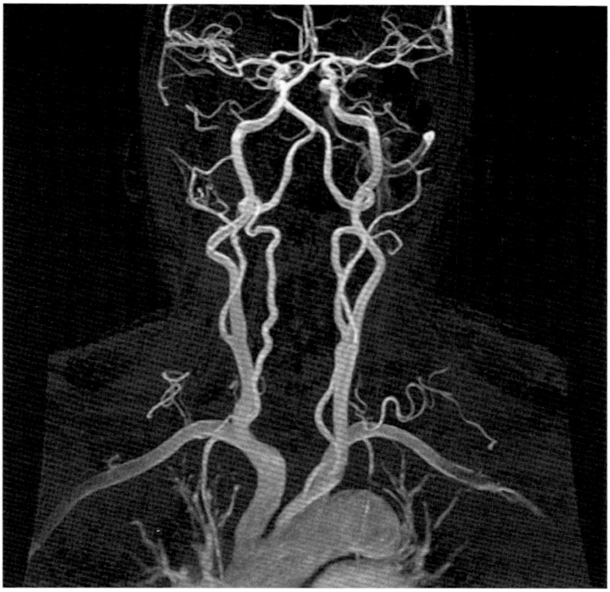

FIGURE 9.3. CE-MRA demonstrating coverage from the aortic arch to the intracranial vessels.

center of k-space is being acquired. There are several ways to ensure this.

- *Bolus tracking*. In its more common manifestation, a series of rapid 2D dynamic images are collected so that the contrast arrival can be visualized (e.g., Siemens' CARE bolus). A 3D scan is then initiated by the operator at the appropriate time. Automatic scan initiation (e.g., GE's Smart Prep) works by continually monitoring the baseline signal in a small volume and triggering a 3D scan when a certain threshold is exceeded. It works well in the abdominal aorta but is less effective in smaller vessels.
- *Test bolus*. A small test dose (2 ml) may be administered to time the arrival of the bolus in the vessel of interest. This then ensures a correct interval is observed for the subsequent real scan using the full dose.

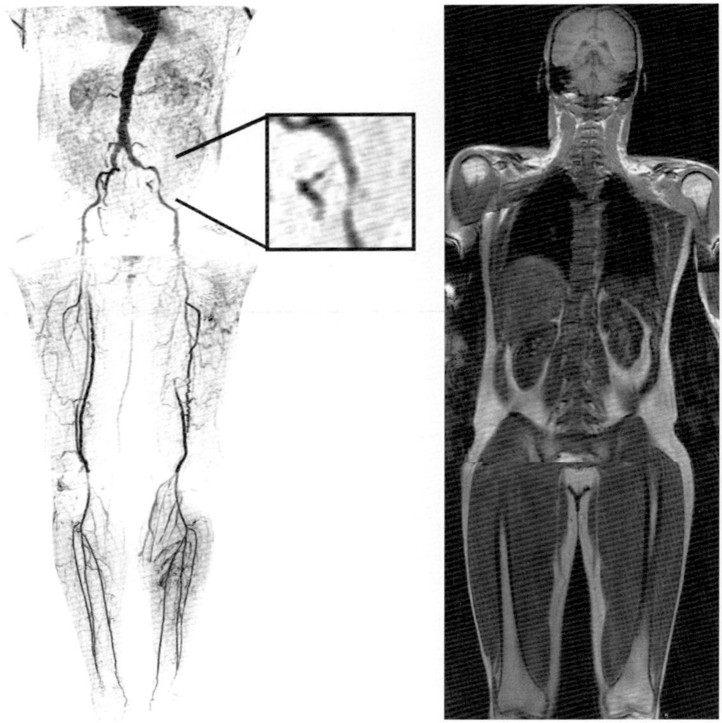

FIGURE 9.4. Examples of a three-station stepping table technique. (left) Peripheral MRA covering the aorto–illiac arteries down to the tibial arteries. (right) Whole-body screening study.

- *Time-resolved MRA.* This method involves imaging with high enough temporal resolution so that the arterial and venous phases of contrast uptake may be separated. TRICKS is an example of this type of sequence and utilizes keyhole imaging to achieve the required temporal resolution (see below).
- *Reordering k-space.* A slightly different approach is to vary the order in which *k*-space data are acquired so that the center of *k*-space (the bulk of the image signal; see Chapter 1) is filled around the time of the arterial phase (e.g., CENTRA).

❖ What is Keyhole Imaging?
This is an example of a partial *k*-space acquisition in order to improve imaging speed. Often used in MRA to ensure good temporal and spatial resolution, it involves acquiring the full *k*-space data once, and then subsequently only the center (or keyhole) of *k*-space is recorded to ensure the contrast changes are represented. The image data at the edges of *k*-space are later "filled in" from the initial scan.

Chapter 10
Musculoskeletal MRI

MRI is arguably the most useful tool in musculoskeletal imaging. Its main strengths lie in its ability to provide diagnostic information in suspected joint disease, bone disease, and assessment of masses involving soft tissue and/or bone. A further advantage lies in the ability to add sequences in any plane depending on the clinical information required.

10.1 KNEE—INTRODUCTION

Internal derangement is the common indication for knee MRI usually caused by traumatic injury in the young or degenerative changes in the elderly. Articular cartilage degeneration in the form of osteoarthritis represents a major cause of morbidity in the adult population of the world. Currently, using specific imaging sequences MRI compares favorably with arthroscopy in the detection of cartilage defects. Other indications for MRI of the knee include suspected infection, osteonecrosis, or tumor imaging.

10.2 CONVENTIONAL TECHNIQUES

Role of MRI

✓ Meniscal degeneration and tears
✓ Anterior/posterior cruciate ligament disruption
✓ Collateral ligaments injury
✓ Chondromalacia patellae
✓ Extensor mechanism abnormalities: patellar tendonitis, patella alta and baja, patella bursae
✓ Ganglion, meniscal and synovial cysts
✓ Fractures
✓ Synovitis

Protocols

- *Image plane*. The sagittal *plane* is good for cruciate ligaments and menisci. The coronal plane is better for detached meniscal fragments, meniscocapsular separation, and collateral ligaments. The patellofemoral joint is best assessed in the axial plane.

> Top Tip! To ensure the anterior cruciate ligament is seen in the sagittal plane the foot may be rotated a few degrees. Alternatively, it may be more comfortable for the patient to maintain his own position and utilize oblique imaging.

- *General imaging*. T_1–*W* images are useful for meniscal and ligamentous imaging. T_2–*W* images are useful for anterior cruciate ligament tears if T_1 images are indeterminate or if fluid is present.

Example sequence: Sagittal SE with TE/TR = 10/600 ms with 3.5 mm thickness, FOV 15–16 cm, 512 × 256 matrix.

- *PD-weighting*. *PD–W* images are useful for meniscal tears (T_2–*W* only shows full tears due to fluid).

Example sequence: Coronal FSE with TE/TR = 14/2660 ms.

- *Fat suppression*. This is used to eliminate the bright fat signal to increase conspicuity of bone marrow, meniscus, and cartilage.

Example sequence: (STIR or similar) inversion recovery FSE with TE/TR = 38 /5040 ms with 3.5 mm thickness, 320 × 256 matrix.

- *Contrast enhancement*. This is helpful in bone tumors to define location, and to determine the nature of the tumor and its suitability for biopsy.
- *Other sequences*. These include state-of-the-art sequences, such as steady-state or driven equilibrium, that offer improved contrast between cartilage and other tissues compared to standard sequences.

Example sequences: SSFP (fat suppression or even water-selective excitation where possible) TE/TR/flip = 8/16 ms/25°.

or

3D-DEFT with fat suppression, TE/TR = 20/300 ms, 3 mm thickness.

RF Coils

Most manufacturers now offer dedicated knee coils usually consisting of a cylindrical configuration, similar to the head coil, to provide a homogeneous imaging volume. Surface coils are also used when the knee joint is too large or the patient is unable to extend the knee to fit in a rigid coil. Small (47 mm) microscopy coils may also be used at high field for optimum resolution.

Example

Figure 10.1 shows a proton density-weighted axial image in a patient with an osteochondral fracture of the medial patella facet and a detached intra-articular fragment (arrow). Note the marrow edema and missing medial patella retinaculum. Surgery confirmed these findings.

10.3 ADVANCED APPLICATIONS

Physiological Loading

Investigation of articular cartilage changes (volume, thickness, and signal intensity) following axial compression is of particular

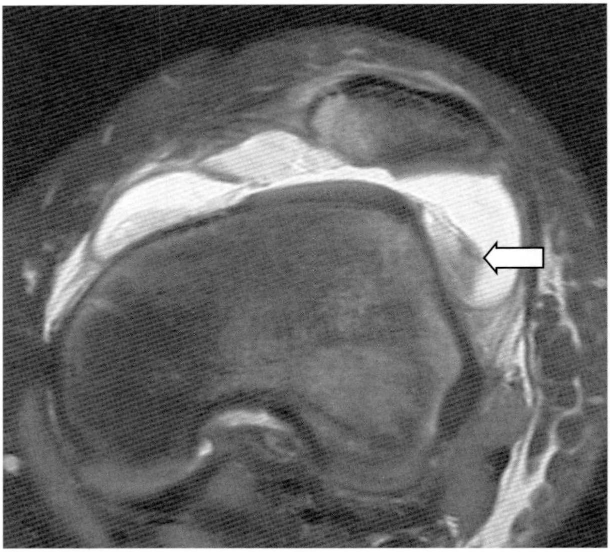

FIGURE 10.1. Axial *PD–W* images in a patient demonstrating a fracture of the medial patella with detached intra-articular fragment (arrow).

interest. Scans are performed prior to and immediately following the application of a physiologically relevant load. This can be accomplished by means of strenuous exercise undertaken outside the magnet or involve the use of MR-compatible devices for in situ compression, permitting a more controlled investigation.

Delayed Contrast and T_1 Mapping

Contrast may be administered and a few hours later the gadolinium penetration into the cartilage can be used to assess glycosaminoglycan content. Several different inversion recovery sequences may be acquired to enable pixel-by-pixel T_1 maps to be calculated demonstrating faster wash-out in diseased cartilage.

High Field

The extra signal-to-noise advantage of high-field MRI is particularly beneficial to orthopedic work for improving the available image detail. Modern scanners can now produce excellent knee images, with in-plane resolutions down to a 200 μm, able to show microtears in ligaments. Trabecular bone, with individual diameters between 50–200 μm is also readily observed at higher field (see Figure 10.2). High-resolution imaging may soon have a role in assisting cellular implantation as treatment for early degeneration of cartilage.

10.4 SHOULDER—INTRODUCTION

Unlike other areas of orthopedic work, shoulder imaging is being increasingly performed by ultrasound. However, MR imaging of the shoulder is commonly performed in rotator cuff disease.

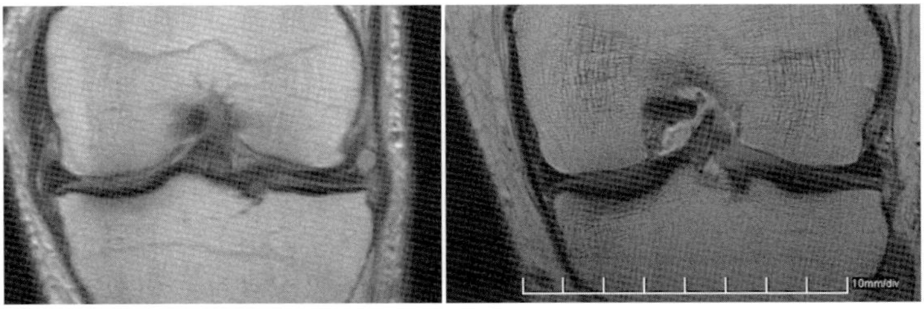

FIGURE 10.2. Coronal images of the knee at 1.5 Tesla (left) and 3.0 Tesla (right), with in-plane resolutions of 0.2 and 0.1 mm^2, respectively. The trabeculae appear thicker at high field due to increased susceptibility effects.

Modern scanners are able to deliver images of clinical quality overcoming the off-center fields of view which are required while maintaining homogeneity. The other main area requiring assessment is shoulder instability. In order to get comprehensive anatomical detail of the glenoid labrum, the biceps anchor, and the glenohumeral ligaments, it is essential to distend the joint. This procedure, termed *MR arthrography*, is usually carried out after instillation of 10–20 cm^3 of saline with a 0.01% concentration of gadolinium under fluoroscopic guidance.

10.5 CONVENTIONAL TECHNIQUES

Role of MRI

- ✓ Evaluation of shoulder pain
- ✓ Conditions affecting the shoulder such as arthritis, bone tumors, infection
- ✓ Shoulder instability/recurrent dislocation
- ✓ Rotator cuff disorders
- ✓ Post-operative assessment

Protocols

- *Positioning*. It is important to keep the arm alongside the body in the neutral position.
- *Coronal*. This includes T_1–W and STIR or T_2–W SE fat suppression or T_2*–W gradient-echo.
- *Sagittal*. This is T_2–W FSE.
- *Axial*. This is proton-density fat suppression, T_2*–W gradient-echo.
- *MR arthrography*. This is T_1 fat suppression in the axial, sagittal, and coronal planes.
- *Post-surgery*. Gradient-echo sequences should be avoided. It is essential to utilize optimized sequences (e.g., FSE-XL) to minimize susceptibility artifacts due to metallic debris from arthroscopy and/or staples from surgical procedures.

> Top Tip! When planning a coronal acquisition, scroll through the upper slices to find the supraspinatus muscle and plan the angle from this.

RF Coils

Usually some general-purpose flexible coil can be used in cases of shoulder imaging although dedicated shoulder coils are also available with separate anterior and posterior coil loops.

10.6 HAND AND WRIST—INTRODUCTION

Over the last few years MRI has become increasingly useful in defining subtle injuries of the hand and wrist. Thanks to improvements in imaging techniques and new coil technology MRI is able to provide the high spatial resolution necessary to visualize the most intricate anatomy of the hand and wrist. Suspected tendon pathology, although seen well on MRI, can be performed dynamically on ultrasound.

10.7 CONVENTIONAL TECHNIQUES

Role of MRI

✓ Ligamentous pathology (scalpholunate, etc.)
✓ Occult fracture
✓ Avascular necrosis
✓ Kienbock's disease
✓ Triangular fibrocartilage complex (TFCC) tears
✓ Rheumatoid disease
✓ Tendon lesions

Protocols

- *Coronal plane.*
- *PD–W or T_2-weighted.* This is fat suppression. FOV 12–15 cm with 512 matrix.
- *T_1-weighted.* This is standard spin-echo.

Example sequence TE/TR 11/500 ms, slice = 3/0.3 mm, 384 matrix, 14 cm FOV.

- *Sagittal and axial.* This is T_2–*W* FSE, T_1–*W*.

RF Coils

A suitable small-volume phased array (e.g., a knee coil) is required to provide the required SNR and resolution. Alternatively, small (3–5 inch diameter) surface coils may be used. Patient positioning may be supine with, space permitting, the hand placed in the coil by the side, or prone, with the hand in front of the head. The latter places the coil at the isocenter, whereas the former is more comfortable but necessitates off-center imaging and a reduction in image quality. Dedicated wrist coils are also available providing a small FOV (12 cm) and adjustable to accommodate the different patient set-ups.

Examples

Figure 10.3 shows two example images of the wrist acquired at 3.0 Tesla in a patient with a ganglion. The image on the left is a

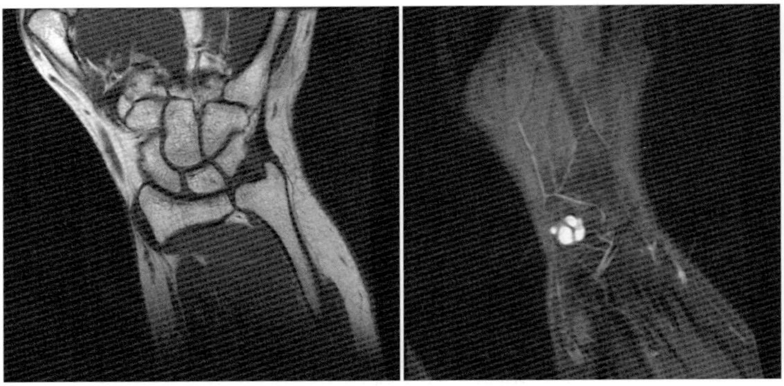

FIGURE 10.3. Example wrist images in a patient. (left) T_1-weighted image shows trabeculae detail and (right) a ganglion is seen in this fat-suppressed image.

T_1-weighted spin-echo sequence and demonstrates the trabeculae. On the right a ganglion can be seen in this STIR sequence.

10.8 ADVANCED APPLICATIONS

Advanced Kinematic RF Coils

New types of wrist coil are being introduced that permit imaging of the wrist over a full range of rotations and movements. Imaging the wrist joint during motion improves the visualization of pathology that may not be seen in a static image.

Dedicated MR Systems

Dedicated extremity scanners now offer a full range of imaging sequences and cover all aspects of musculoskeletal imaging including the shoulder. Typically, operating with a low field (e.g., 0.2 Tesla) permanent magnet, they provide a cheaper alternative to whole-body systems and their siting requirements are substantially easier to accommodate.

10.9 FOOT AND ANKLE—INTRODUCTION

With 26 joints and over a dozen tendons and ligaments careful attention needs to be paid to the provisional diagnosis and main region of interest. It is useful to separate the forefoot as a distinct area and also the ankle and hindfoot as a specific area requiring different imaging planes.

10.10 CONVENTIONAL TECHNIQUES

Role of MRI

- ✓ Ligamentous injury (anterior and posterior talo-fibular, calcaneo fibular)
- ✓ Occult bone injury (Stress fractures)
- ✓ Tendon tears and tendinosis
- ✓ Osteochondral injuries
- ✓ Plantar fasciitis
- ✓ Infection
- ✓ Sinus tarsi syndrome
- ✓ Impingement syndromes (medial, lateral, os-trigonum, etc.)

Protocols

- *Axial*. This includes T_1–*W*, T_2–*W* FSE and is used for assessment of tendons around the ankle joint.
- *Coronal*. This is used for *PD*–*W* or T_2–*W* fat suppression, assessment of talar dome osteochondral injuries, and also medial and lateral impingement syndromes.
- *Sagittal*. Use fat suppression such as STIR to get a bird's-eye view of pathology within the bone framework.

10.11 HIPS—INTRODUCTION

Hip pain is a common symptom and often plain radiographs are normal. The hips are not infrequently involved in a number of pediatric conditions listed below. MRI is used in septic arthritis of the hip for early diagnosis and although ultrasound is reliable in the demonstration of effusions it is often nonspecific. Pigmented villonodular synovitis and synovial chondromatosis also involve the hip and MRI is helpful in detailed assessment. Avascular necrosis of the hip has serious consequences and early diagnosis provides a window of opportunity for surgical core decompression depending on staging. Labral tears are best diagnosed using the technique of MR arthrography. In other sports injuries, MRI allows the elegant demonstration of muscle and tendon strain/tears, particularly the psoas, adductors, and hamstrings. Usually both hips are imaged using a large field of view, but single hip imaging is preferred with a smaller FOV for MR arthrography.

Role of MRI

- ✓ Avascular necrosis
- ✓ Perthes disease
- ✓ Slipped epiphysis

✓ Developmental dysplasia
✓ Arthritis/synovitis
✓ Transient bone marrow edema
✓ Labral tears
✓ Sports injuries
✓ Hip pain of uncertain origin

Protocols

- *Coronal*. This includes T_1–*W* and STIR.
- *Axial*. This includes *PD–W* fat suppression and T_2–*W*.
- *Sagittal*. T_2–*W* is optional.
- *MR arthrography*. This includes T_1–*W* fat suppression in orthogonal planes plus radial images.

Appendix I
Pulse Sequence Acronyms

This section lists over 120 acronyms and abbreviations used to describe, or associated with, MR pulse sequences. A brief explanation is given with each entry.

ASSET Array SenSitive Encoding Technique. GE utilization of parallel imaging.

bFFE Balanced Fast Field Echo. A so-called "true FISP" gradient-echo sequence using balanced rewinding gradients to reset phase at the end of each TR.

CENTRA Contrast ENhanced Timing Robust Angiography. Philips sequence that reorders *k*-space acquisition so that the center of *k*-space data is collected first in order to improve CE-MRA.

CP (CPMG) Carr-Purcell (. . . Meiboom-Gill). Original multiple spin-echo sequence for measuring T_2. Later modified to cycle the direction of the refocusing pulse to improve accuracy.

CHARM CHunk Acquisition and Reconstruction Method. Philips MRA sequence that uses overlapping volumes and a special algorithm to reduce artifacts at the edges of the slabs.

CHESS CHEmical Selective Saturation. Fat suppression technique using a narrow bandwidth RF pulse centered on the fat peak.

CISS Constructive Interference Steady-State. Siemens sequence combining two FISP echoes to give strong T_2-weighting.

CSI Chemical Shift Imaging. Multiple voxel spectroscopy acquisition in which metabolite peaks may be displayed in (usually) color overlaying anatomic images.

CSPAMM Complementary SPAMM. Adaptation to the conventional SPAMM method to improve the visual contrast of the taglines in a spin-tagged cardiac image.

DANTE Delays Alternating with Nutations for Tailored Excitations. Spin-tagging sequence used in cardiac imaging.

DEFAISE Dual Echo Fast Acquisition Interleaved Spin-Echo.

DEFT Driven Equilibrium Fourier Transformation.

DESS Double Echo Steady-State. Combines a FISP and PSIF echo to produce images with large fluid signal for use in orthopedic imaging.

DIET Delayed Interval Echo Train. Use of an increased interval between the first two refocusing pulses of a FSE sequence to produce a more typical spin-echo fat contrast.

DRESS Depth REsolved Surface coil Spectroscopy. Simple MRS acquisition involving excitation of a large volume underneath a surface coil.

DRIVE Philips Driven equilibrium sequence maintaining good T_2-weighting in short scan times.

DTI Diffusion Tensor Imaging.

DWI Diffusion-Weighted Imaging.

DWIBS Philips abbreviation of Diffusion weighted Whole body Imaging with Body background Suppression. Whole-body screening technique.

EPI Echo Planar Imaging. Very fast imaging sequence, acquiring all the necessary image data in a single TR.

FADE Fast Acquisition Dual Echo. Sequence similar to DESS.

FAME Fast Acquisition MultiEcho.

FAST Fourier Acquired Steady-sTate.

FATE FAst Turbo Echo.

FAIR Flow-sensitive Alternative Inversion Recovery. Use of selective and nonselective RF pulses as an arterial spin-labeling method of perfusion imaging.

FE Field Echo. Another term for gradient-echo.

FEDIF Field Echo with the echo time set for water and fat to be out of phase.

FESUM Field Echo with the echo time set for water and fat to be in phase.

FGRE Fast GRadient-Echo.

FGRET Fast GRadient-echo Echo Train. GE sequence combining a gradient-echo with EPI readout to provide very fast images.

FIESTA Fast Imaging Employing steady-STAte. True refocused steady-state sequence.

FISP Fast Imaging with Steady-state Precession. Siemens sequence using phase rewinding gradients. "True FISP" utilizes rewinding gradients in each direction.

FLAIR FLuid Attenuated Inversion Recovery. Use of a very long inversion time to suppress fluid signal.

FLARE Fast Low Angle Recalled Echo. Sequence similar to FLASH.

FLASH Fast Low Angle SnapsHot. Siemens rapid gradient-echo sequence using a small flip angle and short TR.

FSE Fast Spin Echo. Multiple spin-echo sequence with separately phase-encoded echoes to enable image data to be acquired more rapidly.

FSE-XL GE's optimized version, which includes blurring cancellation for improved quality.

FRFSE Fast Recovery FSE, driven equilibrium version of FSE.

FSPGR Fast SPoiled GRadient. GE sequence similar to Turbo FLASH using RF spoiling. Also sometimes denoted as FMPSPGR (MultiPlanar).

GRAPPA GeneRalised Autocalibrating Partially Parallel Acquisition. Parallel imaging technique.

GRASE GRadient- And Spin-Echo sequence. A sequence whereby a train of refocusing pulses and gradient reversals produces mixed spin-echo and gradient-echo contrast.

GRASS Gradient Recalled Acquisition in Steady-State. GE steady-state sequence.

HARP HARmonic Phase method, which permits automated analysis of spin-tagged images in cardiac MRI.

HASTE HAlf Fourier Single shot Turbo spin-Echo. FSE-type sequence in which only half of *k*-space data is acquired to further improve imaging speed.

IPAT Integrated Parallel Acquisition Technique; Siemen's parallel imaging.

IR Inversion Recovery. Use of a 180° excitation pulse to invert spins. Often prefixed on sequences to mean "prepared" with inversion recovery.

ISIS Image Selected In vivo Spectroscopy. Method of MRS localization using both selective and nonselective inversion pulses.

***k–t* BLAST** *k*-space and time-space Broad use Linear Acquisition Speed-up Technique. Exploits the *k*-space and temporal correlations of dynamic data ascertained from low-resolution "training" images (of the heart, for instance). This is then used in subsequent scans to speed up image time.

LAVA Liver Acquisition with Volume Acceleration. GE 3D gradient-echo sequence that uses SPECIAL fat suppression.

MAST Motion Artifact Suppression Technique. A flow-compensated sequence.

MEDIC MultiEcho Data Image Combination. A Siemens sequence with a mixed weighting from the combination of several gradient-echoes.

MEMP MultiEcho MultiPlanar. Old GE term for a multiple spin-echo sequence acquiring more than one slice.

MESS MultiEcho Single Shot.

MOTSA Multiple Overlapping Thin Section Angiograms. Use of several 3D volume acquisitions at high resolution to cover a larger volume in TOF-MRA.

MPGR MultiPlanar GRadient-echo.

MPRAGE Magnetization Prepared Rapid Acquisition by Gradient-Echo. 3D version of turbo-FLASH.

MRSI MR Spectroscopic Imaging (see CSI).

MSE Multiple Spin-Echo.

OOPS Out-Of-Phase Scanning. Deliberately acquiring images with fat–water signal cancellation to improve visualization in certain situations.

PACE Prospective Acquisition CorrEction. A sequence using navigator echoes to reduce motion artifacts.

PEAR Phase Encoded Artifact Reduction. Real-time adjustment of *k*-space acquisition as a method of respiratory gating, used by Philips.

PFI Partial Flip Imaging.

PGSE Pulsed Gradient Spin-Echo. Conventional diffusion-weighted sequence using a positive and negative gradient pair to sensitize the image to microscopic motion.

PILS Parallel Imaging with Localized Sensitivities, similar to SMASH.

POMP Phase Offset MultiPlanar. Speeding up image time by acquiring two slices simultaneously using composite RF pulses.

PRESS Point RESolved Spin-echo. Spectroscopy sequence using three 180° pulses for localization.

PRESTO PRinciples of Echo Shifting with a Train of Observations. Steady-state-based EPI sequence used by Philips.

PROBE PROton Brain Examination. GE spectroscopy acquisition.

PROPELLER Periodically Rotated Overlapping ParallEL Lines with Enhanced Reconstruction. Motion reduction method whereby *k*-space lines are acquired at different angles or "blades".

PROSE PROstate Spectroscopy Examination. GE MRS sequence specifically designed for the prostate with the non-excitation of fat.

PROSET PRinciple Of Selective Excitation Technique. Philips sequence using a binomial pulse for fat or water only excitation.

PS Partial Saturation.

PSIF Reverse of FISP sequence! Pulse sequence is the mirror image of FISP.

QUEST QUick Echo Split-imaging Technique.

RACE Real-time ACquisition and velocity Evaluation. Fast one-dimensional imaging technique for measuring the velocity of blood.

RARE Rapid Acquisition with Refocused Echoes. Generic name for sequences such as FSE, TSE, and so on.

RAM-FAST Rapid Acquisition Magnetization prepared FAST sequence.

REST REgional SaTuration. Saturation bands outside the image volume to remove flow artifacts.

RESTORE Siemens-driven equilibrium sequence.

RISE Rapid Imaging Spin-Echo, same as FSE, and the like.

ROAST Resonant Offset Averaging steady-STate. Term used to describe True FISP sequences with phase-cycled RF pulses to reduce artifacts.

RODEO ROtating Delivery of Excitation Off resonance. Use of narrow RF pulses centered on either fat or water to suppress these signals.

ROPE Respiratory Ordered Phase Encoding. Gating method whereby lines of *k*-space data are acquired at the same point in the respiratory cycle.

SCIC Surface Coil Intensity Correction. GE's post-processing method to remove the B_1 inhomogeneity (GE).

SENSE SENSitive Encoding. Philips implementation of parallel imaging.

SHORT SHOrt Repetition Technique, similar to FLASH.

SMASH SiMultaneous Acquisition of Spatial Harmonics. Parallel imaging method that operates in *k*-space rather than image space like SENSE.
(or) Short Minimum Angle SHot, similar sequence to FLASH.

SPACE Sampling Perfection with Application optimized Contrasts using different flip angle Excitations. A Siemens 3D volume sequence with T_2 contrast.

SPAIR SPectral Attenuated Inversion Recovery. Philips SPIR-based sequence, which uses a variable delay to ensure the fat signal is correctly inverted and the sequence is less sensitive to B_1 inhomogeneity.

SPAMM SPAtial Modulation of Magnetization. Spin-tagging method used in cardiac imaging.

SPECIAL SPECtral Inversion At Lipids. Fat-suppression method using a spectral–spatial inversion pulse at the fat resonance.

SPGR SPoiled GRadient-echo (see also FSPGR).

SPIDER Steady-state Projection Imaging with Dynamic Echo-train Read out. Rapid imaging method whereby k-space is filled in a radial trajectory.

SPIR SPectral saturation with Inversion Recovery. Fat suppression implemented by Philips, which is a combination of frequency selective and T_1 recovery methods.

SS Single-shot, used sometimes to prefix sequences (e.g., ssFSE) which acquire all *k*-space data in one TR.

SSFP Steady-State Free Precession. Sequence similar to FIESTA or TrueFISP.

SSRF Spectral-Spatial Radio Frequency pulses. GE's RF pulses, which do not excite the fat signal.

STAGE Small Tip Angle Gradient-Echo. Similar sequence to FLASH.

STAIR Solution and Tissue Attenuation Inversion Recovery. Use of two differently timed inversion pulses to suppress CSF and fat signal in the brain.

STEAM STimulated Echo Acquisition Mode. Spectroscopy localization method using three 90° pulses.

STIR Short Tau Inversion Recovery. Fat suppression using inversion recovery with a short inversion time (tau).

SVS Single Voxel Spectroscopy.

THRIVE T_1 High Resolution Isotropic Volume Examination. Image sequence (Philips) utilizing SPIR fat suppression and parallel imaging to acquire fast 3D T_1-weighted images in a single breath-hold.

TIM Total Imaging Matrix. Siemens utilization of different coil combinations to provide a 200 cm field of view for whole-body screening.

TIRM Turbo Inversion Recovery Measurement. Similar sequence to FLAIR for producing dark fluid images.

TOF Time Of Flight angiography technique.

TONE Tilted Optimized Nonsaturated Excitation. Time-of-flight MRA technique using a variable flip angle across the imaging slab to reduce saturation effects.

TRAPS TRAnsitions between Pseudo-steady-State. Sequence designed to reduce RF heating at high field strengths.

TRICKS Time Resolved Imaging of Contrast KineticS. GE keyhole imaging technique to acquire high spatial and temporal resolution images for contrast-enhanced MRA.

True FISP See bFFE.

TSE Turbo Spin-Echo. Siemens version of FSE.

Turbo FLASH FLASH sequence with magnetization preparation.

VEMP GE sequence, abbreviation of Variable Echo MultiPlanar.

VENC Velocity ENCoding. This is the maximum velocity that can be encoded by flow-sensitive gradients in a phase-contrast MRA sequence.

VFL Variable FLip angle. Sequence designed to reduce RF heating at high fields.

VIBE Volume Interpolated Body Examination, fast breath-hold sequence used in the abdomen.

VIBRANT Volume Imaging for BReast AssessmeNT. GE sequence designed to shim each breast separately and improve image quality.

VIPR Vastly undersampled Isotropic Projection Reconstruction. Technique for fast 3D volumes with high temporal and spatial resolution used in contrast-enhanced MRA.

VINNIE Velocity ImagiNg iN cInE mode. Dynamically acquired phase-contrast images to quantify blood flow.

VSS Very Selective Slice. Use of up to 10 saturation pulses outside the voxel to acquire spectroscopy with minimal outer volume contamination (GE).

WEFT Water Elimination Fourier Transformation. Water-suppression method for spectroscopy using an inversion pulse of the water peak.

ZIP Zero fill Interpolation Processing. Zero-filling raw data in order to artificially obtain images at higher spatial resolution.

Appendix II
Miscellaneous

A2.1 LIST OF CONTRAST AGENTS

Commercial Name	Generic Name	Chemical Name	Type
Magnevist	Gadopentetate dimeglumine	Gd-DTPA	Extracellular
ProHance	Gadoteridol	Gd-HP-DO3A	Extracellular
Omniscan	Gadodiamide	Gd-DTPA-BMA	Extracellular
Dotarem	Gadoterate meglumine	Gd-DOTA	Extracellular
Gadovist	Gadobutrol	Gd-DO3A-butrol	Extracellular
Angiomark	Gadofosveset	MS-325	Blood pool
MultiHance	Gadobenate dimeglumine	Gd-BOPTA	Blood pool
Gadomer	Gadomer-17	Gd-DTPA-17	Blood pool
Gadolite	Gadolinium zeolite	Gadolinium zeolite	Oral
Lumirem (or Gastromark)	Ferumoxsil	AMI-121	Oral
Magnevist enteral	Gadopentetate dimeglumine	Gd-DTPA	Oral
Endorem (or Feridex)	Ferumoxide	AMI-25	Liver
Primovist (or Eovist)	Gadoxetic acid disodium	Gd-EOB-DTPA	Liver
Teslascan	Mangafodipir trisodium	Mn-DPDP	Liver

A2.2 THE TRANSITION TO HIGH FIELD

As more and more medical centers move from 1.5 Tesla to 3.0 Tesla, it is instructive to compare the two field strengths in the table.

	1.5 Tesla ⇒ 3.0 Tesla
SNR	Up to × 2
T_1	Longer
T_2/T_2^*	Similar
Chemical shift	×2
	Worse artifacts, better fat suppression
Susceptibility	Worse × 2
Contrast agents	Potential for smaller dose
B_1 (RF field)	Poorer penetration and signal homogeneity
RF power (SAR)	×4
Hardware	Fewer RF coils
Safety	No additional risk
	Increased noise
MRS	Increased peak separation
	Improved sensitivity for other nuclei
fMRI	BOLD up to × 4

Appendix III
Screening Form

This is an example of the questions asked as part of our own screening of patients prior to MRI examinations.

	Yes	No	Details
Have you had a MRI scan before?			
Have you ever had a heart pacemaker or defibrillator fitted?			
Have you ever had any heart surgery or valve replacement?			
Have you ever had any operations to your head, eyes, ears, or spine?			
Have you ever had a brain hemorrhage? Do you have an aneurysm clip?			
Have you had any other operations in the last six weeks?			
Have you ever worked with high-speed grinding machinery/lathes?			
Have you ever had an eye injury involving metal fragments?			
We need to know even if the fragment was removed or if it was many years ago.			
Have you ever had any metal fragments in your body? This includes shrapnel injury, body piercing, or sterilization clips.			
Do you have any artificial implanted devices? This includes artificial joints, artificial limbs, pins or plates, stents, filters, bone fixing plates, hydrocephalus shunts, eye implants, and others (please specify)			
Do you have a skin patch (nicotine/hormone patch) or tattoo?			
Do you have any false teeth, hearing aids, metal dental brace, wig?			
Do you have any of the following (if yes, please give details): asthma, inhalers, epilepsy, renal/kidney failure?			
Have you had an injection during an x-ray, scan, or MRI?			
If yes—did you have a reaction to the injection?			
Are you allergic to any medicines?			
What is your weight?			stones

For Female Patients of Child-Bearing Age

Is there any possibility you are pregnant?
Are you breast feeding?
Have you an intrauterine contraception device fitted?

For All Patients

You will need to remove all metallic objects, e.g., watch, jewelery (excluding rings), credit cards, coins. Also remove all items from your pockets.

Index